ROUTLEDGE LIBRARY EDITIONS:
ALCOHOL AND ALCOHOLISM

Volume 2

ALCOHOL AND AGGRESSION

ALCOHOL AND AGGRESSION

Edited by
PAUL F. BRAIN

Routledge
Taylor & Francis Group
LONDON AND NEW YORK

First published in 1986 by Croom Helm

This edition first published in 2024
by Routledge
4 Park Square, Milton Park, Abingdon, Oxon OX14 4RN

and by Routledge
605 Third Avenue, New York, NY 10158

Routledge is an imprint of the Taylor & Francis Group, an informa business

British Library Cataloguing in Publication Data
A catalogue record for this book is available from the British Library

ISBN: 978-1-032-59082-0 (Set)
ISBN: 978-1-032-61050-4 (Volume 2) (hbk)
ISBN: 978-1-032-61097-9 (Volume 2) (pbk)
ISBN: 978-1-003-46198-2 (Volume 2) (ebk)

DOI: 10.4324/9781003461982

Publisher's Note
The publisher has gone to great lengths to ensure the quality of this reprint but points out that some imperfections in the original copies may be apparent.

Disclaimer
The publisher has made every effort to trace copyright holders and would welcome correspondence from those they have been unable to trace.

ALCOHOL AND AGGRESSION

Edited by Paul F. Brain

CROOM HELM
London • Sydney • Dover, New Hampshire

Croom Helm Ltd, Provident House, Burrell Row,
Beckenham, Kent BR3 1AT
Croom Helm Australia Pty Ltd, Suite 4, 6th Floor,
64-76 Kippax Street, Surry Hills, NSW 2010, Australia

British Library Cataloguing in Publication Data

Alcohol and aggression.
1. Alcoholism 2. Aggressiveness (Psychology)
I. Brain, Paul F.
155.2'32 BF575.A3

ISBN 0-7099-0691-9

Croom Helm, 51 Washington Street,
Dover, New Hampshire 03820, USA

Library of Congress Cataloging in Publication Data

Main entry under title:
Alcohol and agression.

1. Alcohol—physiological effect. 2. Aggressiveness (psychology) 3. Violence. I. Brain, Paul F. (DNLM: 1. Aggression—drug effects. 2. Alcohol drinking. 3. Alcohol, ethyl—pharmacodynamics. 4. Alcoholic intoxication—psychology. 5. Alcoholism—psychology. WM 274 A3492)
QP801.A3A35 1986 616.86'1 85-22437

ISBN 0-7099-0691-9

Typeset by Leaper & Gard Ltd, Bristol, England
Printed and bound in Great Britain by
Biddles Ltd, Guildford and King's Lynn

CONTENTS

PREFACE

Behaviour is a superficially easily understood set of phenomena to which the public nowadays has easy and regular access via popular books and television programmes on the activities of both animals and our own species. The actuality is, however, more complex as behaviour may serve a variety of functions, and its control is a consequence of interactions between a mixture of biological, environmental and experience-related factors.

The above reservations apply most strongly in the case of activities we term 'aggression' or 'violence'. Associations between threat or attack and particular factors often seem converted in the public consciousness into established 'causes' of behaviour. This is an unfortunate tendency as the resulting beliefs (one suspects) may influence policy decisions and produce attitudes to particular problems that are not wholly realistic. *Alcohol and Aggression* examines the claimed relationship between drinking and violence, an area in which many members of the public apparently feel there is clear evidence of a simple causal relationship (see the often cited link between drinking and homicide, rape and other expressions of human hostility that occur in our newspapers). The volume is intended to perform the task in a way accessible to the well-informed and intelligent lay person as well as to the interested academic/professional. Indeed, the examination of actual and claimed relationships in this area often overlap two or more areas of competence, hopefully making the text heuristic in the case of the latter type of reader. The book attempts to do this by using a minimum of technical terminology as well as by defining the nature of the phenomena themselves. Such a volume should be of interest to many biologists, medical workers and social scientists. *Alcohol and Aggression* initially provides comprehensive accounts by specialists on: the nature of aggression (by no means as easy a characterised type of activity as is sometimes implied); biochemical, hormonal and neurophysiological events correlated with alcohol application and the expression of such changes in behavioural terms; evidence to be gleaned from (and the questions left unanswered by) behavioural experiments with animals; diverse natures of and the treatment of data on which claims of an involvement of alcohol in human activities that generally receive the label 'violent' are based;

and potential roles of socio-cultural factors in 'alcohol-related aggression'.

The above accounts all essentially examine (from a variety of perspectives) the recurrent media claim that alcohol causes a percentage of the aggression we see in our everyday lives. A concluding synthesis places the accounts in context, and suggests that the question 'Does alcohol cause aggression?' is itself grossly over-simplistic. It is clear that aggression is not a single attribute, the physiological and biochemical consequences of exposing a living organism to alcohol are extremely involved (depending on, for example, species, strain, dose, prior experiences and time for their expression), and the relating of these biological changes to behaviour (of which aggression is often a minor component) is a most difficult task. Indeed, some of the claimed associations in humans have problems apparently unique to our species. These confusing factors, rather than being causes of concern, should give direction to attempts to express the true complexity of these associations. It is argued that cross-disciplinary approaches which attempt to take into account many types of consideration and resist easy transmutation to simple cause - - - → effect models, provide the way forward in this important area.

It is hoped that this book will provide a timely and well-balanced account of the available data. The intention is to give the reader (irrespective of his/her predispositions) an honest evaluation of the problems inherent in attempts to relate alcohol ingestion to acts (or feelings) of aggression. Improved understanding will hopefully translate eventually into a clearer statement from science and fewer lurid journalistic claims. One must seriously doubt that the elimination of alcohol from soccer grounds will remove a major pharmacological effect on hooliganism, but it may change the participant's lifestyle, destroy a self-excuse and eliminate some potential weapons. In such areas, the clarification of mythologies may be as important as the development of predictive techniques.

Cheers!

Paul F. Brain
Swansea

(the day on which the college was invaded by an Animal Right's group complaining about experiments with alcohol on the basis that they already 'knew' the effects)

LIST OF CONTRIBUTORS

Badawy, Abdulla A.-B., BPharm, PhD, MRC Path.
South Glamorgan Health Authority
Addiction Unit Research Laboratory
Whitchurch Hospital
Cardiff CF4 7XB
Wales
Berry, Michael S., BSc, MSc, PhD
Biomedical and Physiological Group,
Department of Zoology
University College of Swansea
Swansea SA2 8PP
Wales
Brain, Paul F., BSc, PhD
Biomedical and Physiological Group,
Department of Zoology
University College of Swansea
Swansea SA2 8PP
Wales
Coid, Jeremy, MRC Psych, MPhil.
Senior Registrar in Forensic Psychiatry
The Maudsley Hospital
Denmark Hill
London SE5
England
Evans, Charles M., BSc, PhD
Department of Physiology
The Medical School
Vincent Drive
University of Birmingham
Birmingham B15 2TJ
England
Smoothy, Robert, BSc PhD
Biomedical and Physiological Group,
Department of Zoology
University College of Swansea
Swansea SA2 8PP
Wales

1 THE NATURE OF AGGRESSION

Paul F. Brain

Introduction

It must first be emphasised that *aggression* is a concept (i.e. a device enabling us to make sense of the complex relationships of our world) *not* an entity. Aggression cannot be measured in any direct sense, and although we often assume that aggressive acts are driven by a motivation (aggressiveness), this is a tautology. One must also stress that it seems inappropriate to many workers to attempt to study so-called 'aggression' in isolation from the rest of behaviour — aggression often accounts for only a small proportion of an individual's activities. There is, in relation to this, some support for the use of the term *agonistic behaviour* which reasonably includes attack as only a part of a continuum of conflict behaviours which also takes in threat, submission, defeat and flight.

Aggression means different things to different people. Indeed, some workers[1] dismiss is entirely, preferring *coercive power* (the property of an activity to force conspecifics to give way). Barnett[2] somewhat whimsically defines aggression as 'a word of many meanings and a source of much confusion'. Part of his complaint is that aggression and violence are used in both popular and scientific writing — making precise definition difficult. We may cynically suggest that aggression is the type of activity that other less reasonable individuals direct towards us — we are 'competitive' or 'simply defending our rights' — they are 'aggressive', 'violent', and indulge in 'acts of terrorism'. Some indication of the current state of confusion is indicated by Van der Dennen,[3] who has compiled a list of 106 definitions of aggression of astounding variability.

A scientifically acceptable definition of aggression is going to constitute a real problem. One useful view of such activities is that proposed by Buss,[4] namely that it is 'the attempt to deliver noxious stimuli (whether or not that attempt is successful)'. Noxious stimuli are seen as physical and/or psychological factors. Workers at various times have claimed that actions should be termed aggression when:

(a) actual or potential noxious stimuli are directed towards some object (generally a conspecific; NB there is considerable debate about the status of predatory responses where the objects are members of other species);
(b) the act is intentional (not accidental) or is perceived as such (NB the considerable difficulties of establishing intentionality in infra-human animals);
(c) the director of the stimuli is emotionally aroused (see Figure 1.1). Although external appearance gives us some clues about an animal's internal state, the science has not advanced much since Darwin's classic observations of 1872 in *The Expression of the Emotions in Man and Animals.*[5] There are also considerable difficulties associated with glib analogies, the powers of humans to disguise true emotions and the fact that most individuals would not eliminate the 'passionless' activities of psychopaths from the category of aggression; and
(d) The 'victim' is motivated to remove itself or avoid such exposure (otherwise sado-masochism and the use of love darts by courting snails would have to be included in such phenomena).

Not all authorities are agreed that aggression needs all four criteria. A vast variety of specialists study aggression from a large number of viewpoints, they are said by Moyer[6] to include anatomists, anthropologists, biochemists, biologists, dentists, ecologists, electro-encephalographists, endocrinologists, ethologists, geneticists, medics, neurologists, pharmacologists, physiologists, primatologists, psychiatrists, psychologists and sociologists, as well

Figure 1.1: Emotional Arousal in a Male Cat in Response to a Conspecific Male; NB the Threat, Piloerection and Direction of the Animal's Weapons of Offence (Teeth and Claws in this Case)

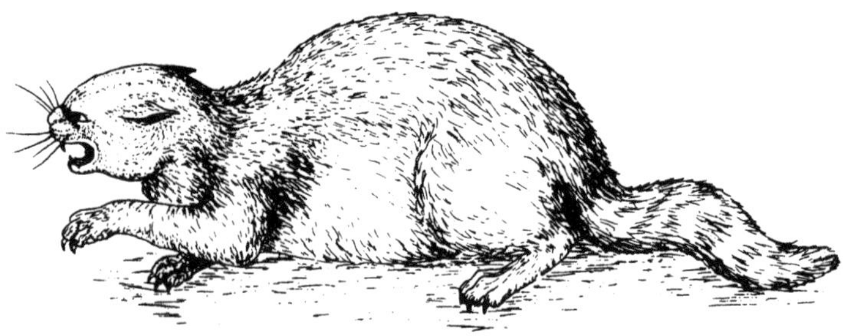

as proponents of cross disciplinary fields, e.g. clinical endocrinologists, experimental therapeutists, neuroendocrinologists, neuropharmacologists, neurophysiologists, neuropsychiatrists, physiological psychologists, physiological zoologists, psychopharmacologists, experts in psychosomatic medicine, social psychologists and sociobiologists. This diversity predictably leads to enormous confusion, especially as even the terminologies differ. One of the problems is that, whereas sociologists and some medical scientists see aggression as an essentially negative characteristic, to be 'cured', most biologists point to the utilities of such behaviour in many animal species. Note also that many social scientists and biologists have very different ways of studying this phenomenon. Is it perhaps best to look at animal and human aggression separately, as the descriptive language and types of study tend to be very different?

Animal Aggression

Biologists argue that intraspecific (between members of the same species) fighting may serve to select breeding individuals as in Red deer (*Cervus elephus*) — see Figure 1.2.

Figure 1.2: The Red Deer Stag Uses the Seasonally Grown Antlers in Generally Non-injurious Encounters in Rutting to Obtain a Harem of Females. Bellowing Serves as a Threat

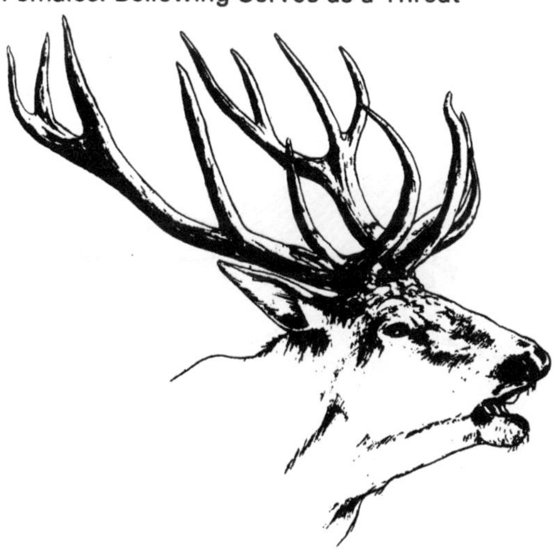

Aggression may also be used to defend an exclusive breeding area by individuals, pairs or groups (a territory) which also has a sexual selection value. This is evident, for example, in the European robin (*Erithacus rubecula*) as in Figure 1.3.

Figure 1.3: Territorial Attack by a Male Robin on a Red-chested Model; NB Red Serves as a Sign Stimulus for Attack and Bird Song in This Situation May be Employed as Territorial Defence

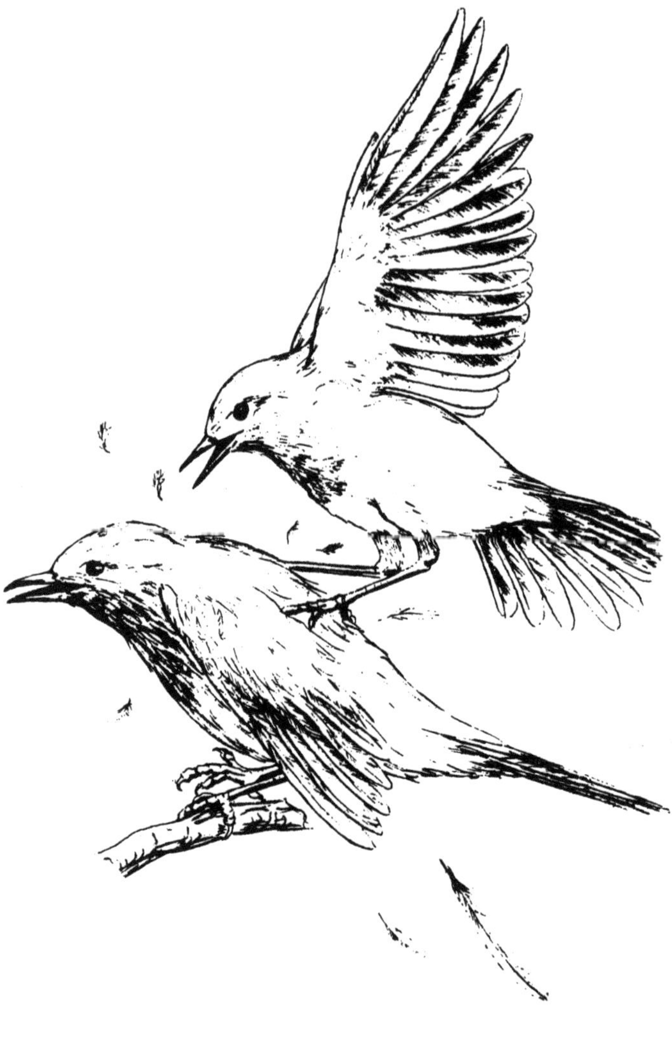

'Aggression' may also be used to develop social organisations. For example, chickens (*Gallus gallus domesticus*) form peck-orders (linear hierarchies) in which there is a chain of dominance where birds may peck with impunity individuals ranked below them, but receive pecks from higher ranking subjects. 'Dominants' consequently have preferred access to limited resources (e.g. food, mates and shelter) in times of shortage, a factor of *obvious* survival value (see Figure 1.4).

Not all hierarchies are linear. Wolves (*Canis lupus*) have complex social organisations (hunting packs) which are said to be maintained by social conflict (see Figure 1.5).

The signals involved in established social organisations may be very subtle. For example, in primates such as Squirrel monkeys (*Saimiri sciureus*) stare threat may be the predominant activity (see Figure 1.6).

Workers with animals generally currently acknowledge that there is no single motivation for aggression.[7] Recent data on rats (*Rattus norvegicus*) and mice (*Mus musculus*) suggest that attack may have a number of different functions even in a single species.

Figure 1.4: The Peck Order in Chickens. The Dominant Bird (right) Simply has to Threaten the Subordinate in Order to Obtain the Resource. Established Hierarchies Show *Social Inertia* with Little Overt Fighting

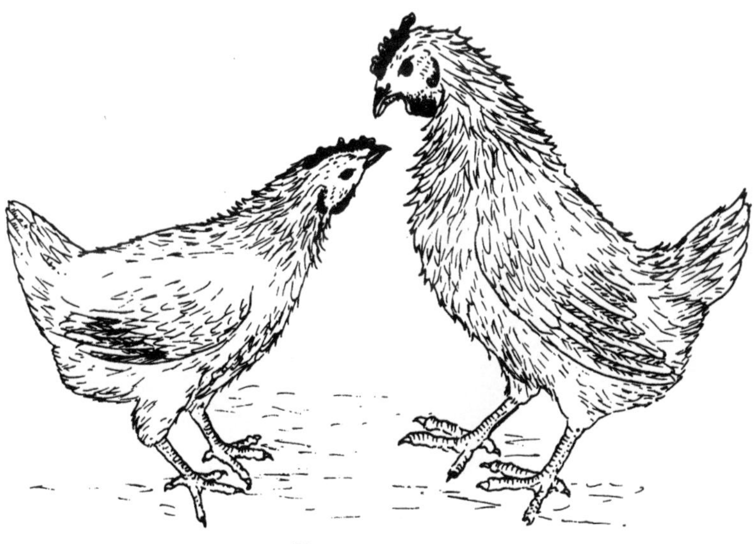

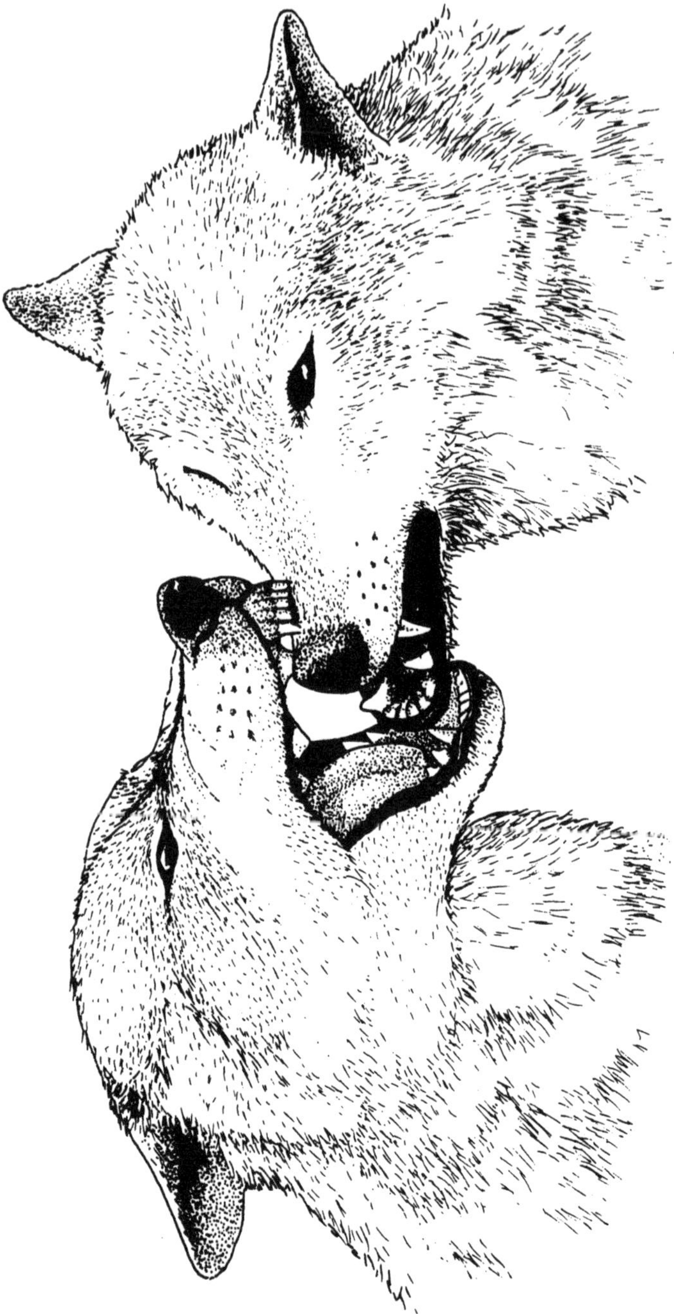

Figure 1.5: The Dominant (left) Wolf Threatens and the Subordinate Exposes his Vulnerable Neck in So-called Ritualised Submission

Figure 1.6: Stare Threat in Two Male Squirrel Monkeys Towards a Member of the Same Species

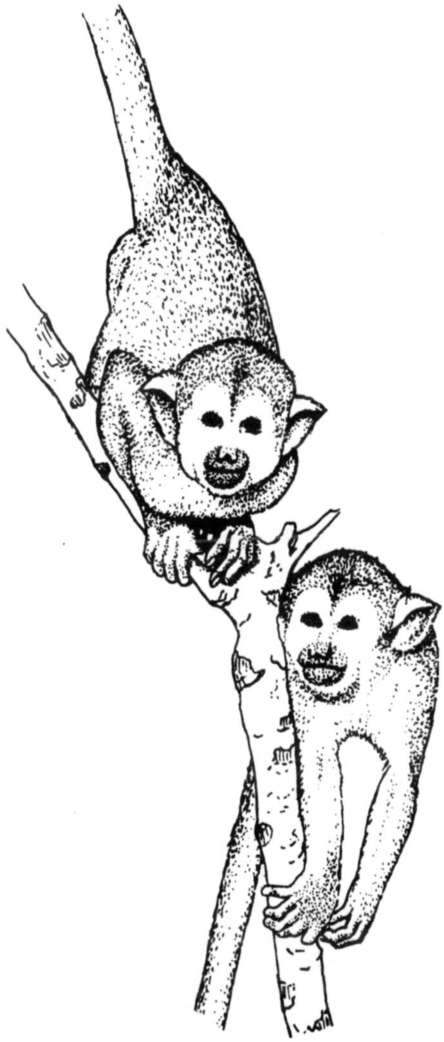

These may include defence, offence and predation (see account in Chapter 8). For example, intermale fighting in feral (wild) rats (see Figure 1.7) is very different to the essentially *defensive* behaviour induced in laboratory rats by exposure to non-avoidable electroshock (see Figure 1.8).

Figure 1.7: Attack by a Territorial Male Rat (right) on an Intruding Male

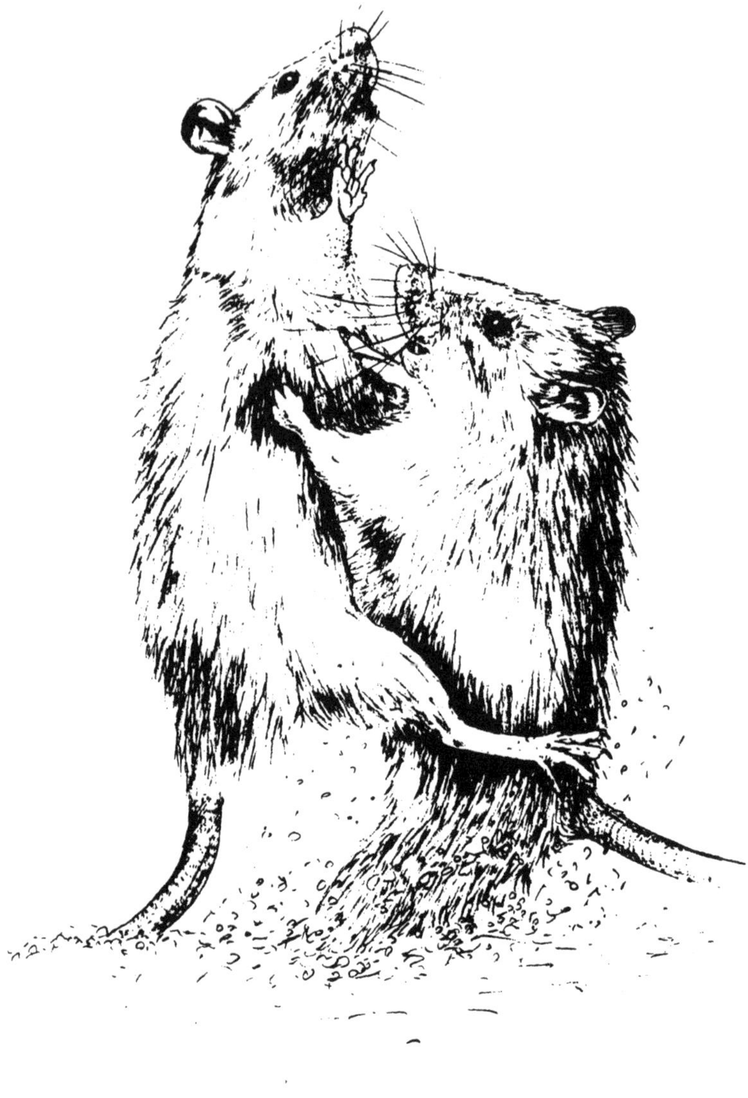

Figure 1.8: Electroshock-induced 'Boxing' in Rats — Said by Blanchard and Blanchard[8] to be Essentially a Defensive Response

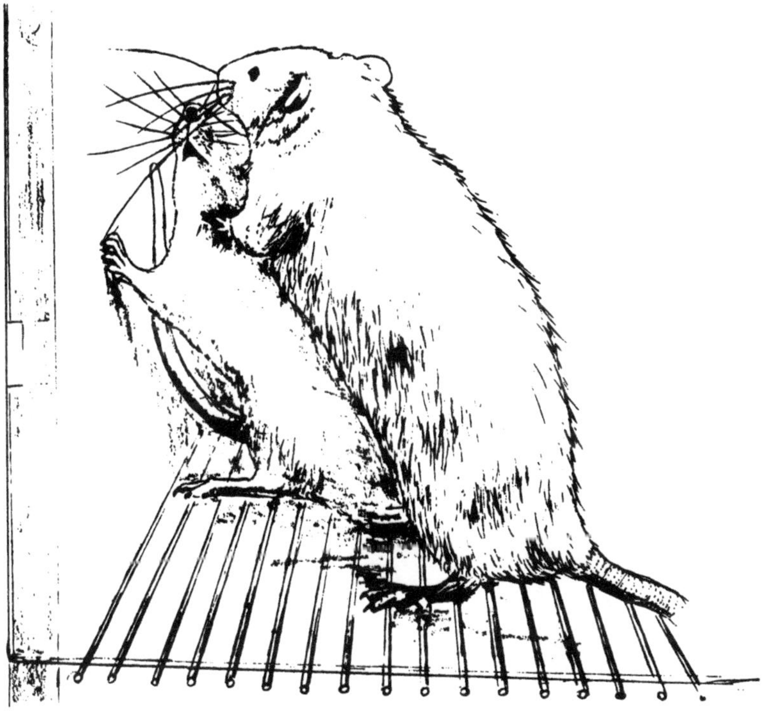

Brain[9] suggests, on the basis of studies involving changing situational, physiological and experiential variables and assessing the bite targets employed (see Figure 1.9), that aggression in infrahumans is usefully divided into:

(1) *Social conflict* — essentially intraspecific competitive behaviour which, if successful, maximises fitness (see the Game Theory considerations of Maynard Smith and Price [10]) and can involve competition for mates, territory or social status. For example, such behaviour can be induced in laboratory mice of some strains by individual housing or reproductive experience.[11] This form of attack evidences an avoidance of directing bites to the vulnerable head and ventral surfaces of the conspecific target animal.

Figure 1.9: Bite Targets Used in a Number of Types of 'Aggression Test' Involving Laboratory Mice

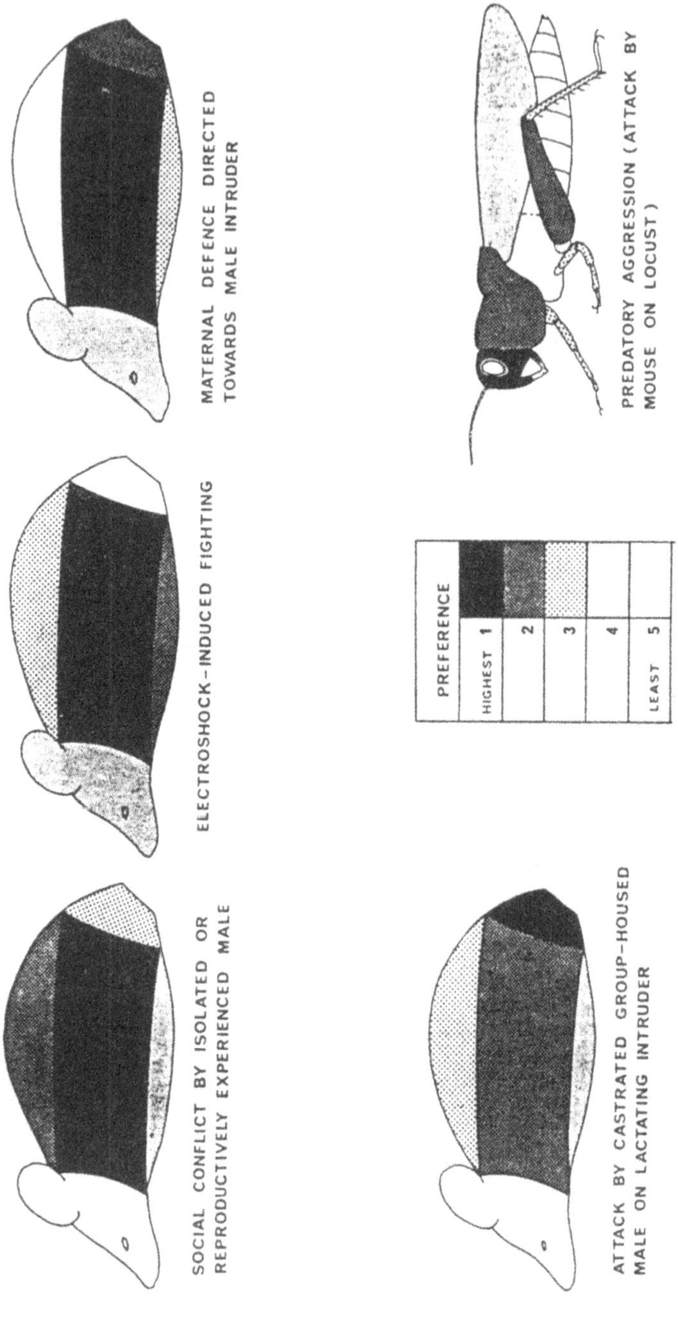

Although dominance is usually a characteristic of males, females of some species may dominate males at most times. For example, female Golden hamsters (*Mesocricetus auratus auratus*) are larger than males and only tolerate them when in oestrus (see Figure 1.10). Also *intact*, female and castrated male resident mice of some strains attack lactating female intruders.

(2) *Parental Defence* — this behaviour seems to be employed to protect offspring, eggs or nest sites. For example, lactating female mice in the presence of their offspring and the absence of their mates attack intruding male conspecifics[12] or even rats.[13] Such activities involve no attempt at injury limitation.

(3) *Electroshock-induced Attack* — which seems in some species, a 'fear'-motivated, self-defensive response. This, however, may not be true of mice.[14] Superficially similar behaviours may also be evident in cornered subordinate animals in social encounters.

Figure 1.10: Typical Social Conflict in *Female* Golden Hamsters; NB the Combatants Use Their Dark Chest Patches in Threat Displays

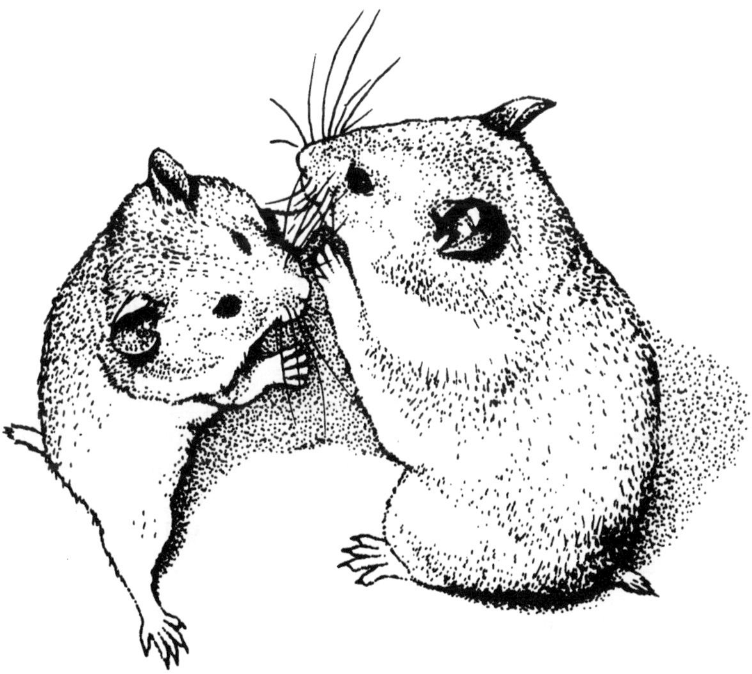

Other forms of 'aggression' have been studied in laboratory rodents. They include *predatory aggression* such as the muricide (mouse-killing) response of rats[15] and locust-killing in mice.[16] There are, however, considerable doubts about the motivations underlying such activities — predation and feeding seem more likely descriptions than aggression. Reproduction termination (pup-killing) in mice has been used as a model of aggression.[17] The genesis of this behaviour is uncertain, it could be impaired maternal activity or a device for recycling resources in the absence of optimal breeding conditions.

Human Aggression

In man, physiology *and* behaviour are much influenced by prior experience, and we are adept in both symbol manipulation and substitution. This gives humans an enormous range of aggression-provoking and aggression-inhibiting stimuli. We are also 'trained' to accept *appropriate* circumstances for aggressive responses, and are conditioned to give 'reasonable' responses in different circumstances. What is sport in one situation becomes assault and battery in others. Naturally, what is or is not viewed as 'aggression' is much influenced by the early conditioning of the observer. Overt expressions of aggression in man are less predictable than those seen in more lowly species.

There are a wide range of views concerning the nature and origins of aggression in man — which is another problem for the scientific study of this phenomenon which are dealt with in detail by Baron,[18] Kutash *et al.*[19] and Van der Dennen,[3] but are briefly:

(a) The Psychoanalytical View of Human Aggression

One of Freud's[20] views of aggression was that it stemmed from an innate, self-directed death wish (thanatos) that could be relieved by redirection towards others (catharsis). One should note that, although this hypothesis currently receives little direct support, the view seems to survive in some popularised writings on aggression.[18]

(b) Aggression viewed as an Instinctive Drive

Classical ethologists such as Lorenz[21] have suggested that aggression is derived from an innate fighting instinct which is common to all animals (including man). Such a view has obvious parallels with Freud's view (given below), and seems a consequence of Lorenz's exposure to the writings of the 'father of psychoanalysis'. One should note that such a completely intrinsic view of the genesis of human aggression meets with little unqualified support by modern ethologists. Much of the criticism of the instinct view of human aggression has been marshalled by Montagu.[22]

(c) Aggression as a Biologically Useful Strategy

Eibl-Eibesfeldt[23] has stressed that fighting may be selected independently by particular species to serve particular roles (usually he feels, related to 'spacing'). He argues that aggression may represent a useful strategy in the obtaining of mate-selection and territory formation. Consequently, species could independently arrive at similar usages — the fact that one gets similar physiological correlates in different species could be due to common selection pressure (especially if the behaviour has to be related to sex or season). This hypothesis does not necessarily view aggression as being genetically transmitted in the way that Lorenz's earlier view did.

(d) Aggression as the Product of Elicited 'Drive' — The Frustration Aggression Hypothesis

One historically influential view of aggression suggested was that it stemmed primarily from an externally elicited 'drive' to harm others. The frustration-aggression hypothesis[24] which suggests that frustration elicits a persistent 'drive' toward aggression is the most influential statement in this framework. Such behaviour is said to be inhibited by fear of punishment, but the instigation is said to remain in these cases and often lead to assaults against secondary targets (including inanimate objects). Secondary targets are regarded as being associated with lower degrees of inhibition than the initial sources of frustration — this has been referred to as 'displaced aggression'.[25]

(e) The Negative Affect-Aggression Hypothesis

This view of aggression has been championed by Baron.[18] He maintains that moderately uncomfortable/stressful situations potentiate attack whereas markedly adverse conditions predispose the organism towards flight. Aggression is in this scheme clearly a coping response.

(f) Aggression as a Learned Social Response

This view is closest to the view of many sociologists and social psychologists of aggression. For example, Bandura[26] has studied the effects of imitation on attack on inflatable 'Bobo' dolls. He feels that a thorough understanding of aggression will be obtained only through careful attention to:

(i) the way in which such behaviour is acquired;
(ii) the factors that instigate the occurrence; and
(iii) the conditions that maintain performance.

In humans, instrumental conditioning and social modelling are clearly strongly involved in the acquisition of responses that receive the label aggression. The former process generally involves acts of aggression being followed by various forms of positive reinforcement, e.g. possession of money, status or toys. The latter phenomenon involves observation of the actions and the outcomes of such actions in others, followed by imitation. Different factors may instigate the occurrence of attack and a variety of conditions, e.g. the obtaining of material or social reinforcers may preserve the strengths of these activities within individual behavioural hierarchies.

General Comments

The diversity of views of the genesis of human aggression strongly suggest that it will be difficult to assess the claimed relationship between alcohol ingestion and violence. Individuals are viewed on instinctive and 'drive' views of aggression as being impelled to attack by internal forces or by external stimuli. In contrast, the strategy and social-learning views suggest that 'violence' occurs at least in part because of learned associations between aggression and environmental factors. The fact that none of these views appears to offer a complete explanation of the genesis of human aggression is due to the fact that such behaviours are heterogeneous (see below) and are products of interaction between biology, situational determinants and experience (see later).

To an even greater degree than in animals, aggression is a term applied in humans to a great range of activities, many of which are likely to have little in common (see Table 1.1). The list is simply intended to show the extreme diversity of individuals and situations which are/have been regarded as appropriate in aggression studies. It should be immediately apparent that the categories show consider-

Table 1.1: The Diversity of Situations in which Human 'Aggression' is Studied

Subjects	Possible sub-divisions	Examples
Sub-adults		Studies on social organisation in pre-school play and nursery groups, individuals in summer camps etc.
Students or 'volunteers' in contrived laboratory situations	Use of provocator	Deliberate antagonism of subject in a 'learning' situation
	Use of questionnaires	Buss-Durkee hostility inventory
	Use of 'hostility' machine (see Figure 1.11)	Choice of 'shock' level delivered to a target
Various tribes	'aggressive' versus 'pacifist' groups	Quolla Indians, !Kung
Participants in hazardous 'field' situations	—	Genoves[27] raft experiments
Military personnel and other occupants of 'war' zones	Combatant Non-combatant	Sniping, bombing, etc. 'Stress' of being 'victims' of war
Sportsmen and sportswomen	Winners/losers	Personality traits of ice hockey players and boxers
Spectators of sports	—	Football 'hooliganism'
Criminal populations	Impulsive versus premeditated and sexual versus non-sexual	Rape, child molesting, homicide and mugging
Drug abusers	Legalised and illegal drugs	use of alcohol, marihuana
'Victims' of crime	—	defence of person or property
Clinical populations	Largely somatic disorders	E.g. persons with endocrine disorders or brain tumours
	Largely psychiatric disorders	manic/depressives, schizophrenics etc

able overlap and whether an action is rated as 'aggressive' can vary with respect to third party observers.

Buss[28] has suggested that human aggressions can be classified on three dichotomies namely whether the act is physical/verbal; active/passive and direct/indirect. This gives a total of eight types of response (see Table 1.2). One should note that many human situations which are said to involve aggression have no obvious animal parallels and generate different conclusions from studies on infra-humans. For example, Buss's hostility machine (see Figure 1.11), which assesses a person's willingness to apparently deliver painful electric shocks to a colleague of the experimenter, suggests that females are more aggressive than males, and that college undergraduates are only slightly less aggressive than psychopaths.

Assessing the Influence of Alcohol on Aggression

Most workers recognise that activities receiving the label 'aggression' are a consequence of subtle interactions between biological, situational and experiential factors. Postulating uniquely biological 'controls' of such activities (especially in humans) is crude as the above factors are not easily separable. The remainder of this volume examines how studies of ethanol's effects on

Table 1.2: A Classification of Human Aggression Based on the Three Dichotomies[28]

Type of aggression	Examples
Physical — active — direct	Stabbing, punching or shooting
Physical — active — indirect	Setting a booby trap or hiring an assassin
Physical — passive — direct	Physically preventing an individual from obtaining a desired goal or performing a desired act (as in picketing)
Physical — passive — indirect	Refusing to perform necessary tasks (e.g. refusal to move during a sit-in)
Verbal — active — direct	Insulting or derogating another person
Verbal — active — indirect	Spreading malicious rumours or gossip about another individual
Verbal — passive — direct	Refusing to speak or answer questions
Verbal — passive — indirect	Failing to make specific verbal comments (e.g. not speaking up in another person's defence when he or she is unfairly criticised)

Figure 1.11: Buss's Hostility Machine

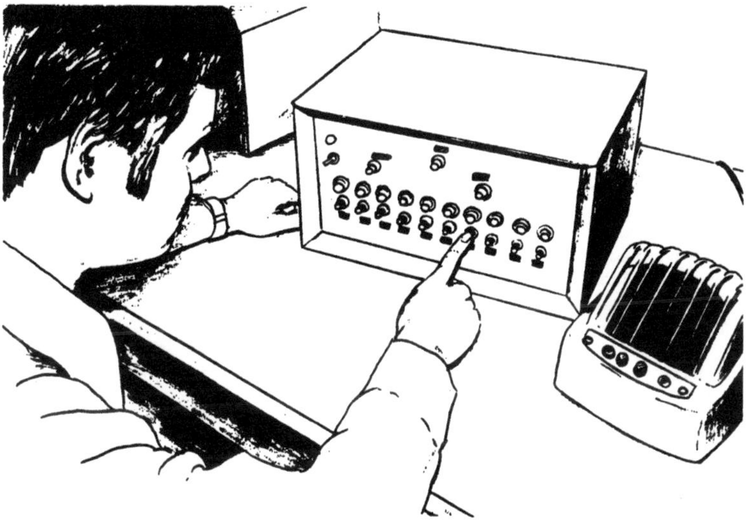

physiology and behaviour in a wide range of species is finally revealing the true complexity of the claimed association between alcohol ingestion and aggression. The resulting picture is considerably more complex than the abolitionist's view that this 'evil of drink' is well established. As well as illustrating the difficulties of the current literature, it is hoped that this book will serve as a spur for research rather than pontification in this area.

References

1. Tedeschi, J.T., Melburg, V. and Rosenfeld, P. 'Is the concept of aggression useful?' in *Multidisciplinary Approaches to Aggression Research* (eds Brain, P.F. and Benton, D.), Amsterdam: Elsevier/North Holland, 1981, pp. 23-38.

2. Barnett, S.A. *Modern Ethology*, Oxford: OUP, 1981.

3. Van der Dennen, J.M.G. 'Problems in the concepts and definitions of aggression, violence and some related terms', *Publication of the Rijksuniversiteit Groningen*, Polemologisch Instituut, The Netherlands, 1980.

4. Buss, A.H. 'Aggression pays' in *The Control of Aggression and Violence* (ed. Singer, J.L.), New York: Academic Press, 1971, pp. 7-18.

5. Darwin, C. *The Expression of the Emotions in Man and Animals*, London: D. Appleton & Company, 1872.

6. Moyer, K.E. 'The need for a new journal', *Aggressive Behavior*, 1974, *1*, preface.

7. Moyer, K.E. 'Kinds of aggression and their physiological basis', *Communications in Behavioral Biology*, 1968, *2*, 65-87.
8. Blanchard, R.J. and Blanchard, D.C. 'Aggressive behavior in rats', *Behavioral Biology*, 1977, *21*, 197-224.
9. Brain, P.F. 'Differentiating types of attack and defense in rodents' in *Multidisciplinary Approaches to Aggression Research* (eds Brain, P.F. and Benton, D.), Amsterdam: Elsevier/North Holland, 1981, pp. 53-78.
10. Maynard Smith, J. and Price, G.R. 'The logic of animal conflict', *Nature* (London), 1973, *246*, 15-18.
11. Brain, P.F., Benton, D. and Bolton, J.C. 'A comparison of agonistic behavior in individually housed male mice and those cohabiting with females', *Aggressive Behavior*, 1978, *4*, 201-6.
12. Al-Maliki, S., Brain, P.F., Childs, G. and Benton, D. 'Factors influencing maternal attack on conspecific intruders by lactating female. "TO" strain mice', *Aggressive Behavior*, 1980, *6*, 103-17.
13. Poshivalov, V.P. 'Inversion of interspecies relations: isolated mice attack rats', *Journal of Higher Nervous Activity*, 1977, *27*, 1316-18.
14. Brain, P.F., Al-Maliki, S. and Benton, D. 'Attempts to determine the status of electroshock-induced attack in laboratory mice', *Behavioural Processes*, 1981, *6*, 171-89.
15. Karli, P. 'The Norway rat's killing response to the white mouse: an experimental analysis', *Behaviour*, 1956, *10*, 81-103.
16. Brain, P.F. and Al-Maliki, S. 'A comparison of "intermale fighting" in "standard opponent" tests and attack directed towards locusts by 'TO' strain mice: effects of simple experimental manipulations', *Animal Behaviour*, 1978, *26*, 723-37.
17. Gandelman, R. and Vom Saal, F.S. 'Pup-killing in mice: the effects of gonadectomy and testosterone administration', *Physiology and Behavior*, 1975, *20*, 252-60.
18. Baron, R.A. *Human Aggression: Perspectives in Social Psychology*, New York: Plenum Press, 1977.
19. Kutash, I.L., Kutash, S.B., Schlesinger, L.B. and Associates, (eds) *Violence: Perspectives on Murder and Aggression*, San Francisco: Jossey-Bass, 1978.
20. Freud, S.A. *General Introduction to Psychoanalysis*, New York: Boni & Liveright, 1920.
21. Lorenz, K. *On Aggression*, New York: Harcourt, Brace & World, 1966.
22. Montagu, A. *Man and Aggression*, second edn (ed. Montagu, A.), London: Oxford University Press, 1973.
23. Eibl-Eibesfeldt, I. 'Evolution of destructive aggression', *Aggressive Behavior*, 1977, *3*, 127-44.
24. Dollard, J. Doob, L. Miller, N. Mourrer, O.H. and Sears, R.R. *Frustration and Aggression*, New Haven, Conn: Yale University Press, 1939.
25. Miller, N.E. 'Theory and experiment relating psychoanalytical displacement to stimulus-response generalization', *Journal of Abnormal and Social Psychology*, 1948, *43*, 155-78.
26. Bandura, A. *Aggression: A Social Learning Analysis*, Englewood Cliffs, NJ: Prentice Hall, 1973.
27. Genoves, S. Acali, Ra 1 and Ra 2 'Some conclusions and hypotheses concerning human friction under isolation and stress, with special reference to intelligence and personality assessment', *Aggressive Behavior*, 1977, *3*, 163-72.
28. Buss, A.H. 'Aggression pays' in *The Control of Aggression and Violence* (ed. Singer, J.L.), New York: Academic Press, 1971, pp. 7-18.

2 NEUROPHYSIOLOGICAL AND ENDOCRINOLOGICAL CONSEQUENCES OF ALCOHOL

Michael S. Berry and *Paul F. Brain*

Introduction

The nervous system and the endocrine system represent the two major coordinating processes of complex multi-cellular animals. Alcohol can influence virtually every aspect of this complex and highly integrated portion of the organism, and those influences account for most of the associated behavioural changes. It consequently seems useful in considering the thesis of this book to sketch the complexities of those systems and to broadly indicate some of the more striking effects of alcohol on neurophysiology and endocrine function.

An early distinction was made between the coordinating role(s) of the neural system and the endocrine glands based on the general features listed in Table 2.1. This still has some validity.

Although there are many exceptions to these below categorisations, and processes often involve both neural and hormonal components (e.g. the adrenal medulla is largely activated by the splanchnic nerve, and many steroid hormones are neurally concentrated and exert effects on neuronal firing), the distinctions at least emphasise that coordination involves more than one kind of message and that slower, more diffuse and more chronic coordination is likely to involve hormones. A number of authorities favour the view that there is a single *neuroendocrine coordinating system*

Table 2.1: Some of the General Features Which are Said to Distinguish Neural and Endocrine Coordination

	Neural	Endocrine
Speed of Reaction	Rapid	Slower
Specificity of Action	Point to Point	Diffuse
Duration of Effects	Acute	Chronic
Variety of Messages	Small	Large

in which different aspects may be accentuated. The intimate relationship between the brain and the endocrine glands is clearly illustrated in many of the more recent accounts. For ease of treatment, however, we will arbitrarily discuss alcohol's influences on neurophysiology before turning to the involvement of this drug in hormonal changes.

Alcohol and Neurophysiology

Alcohol is perceived as exerting its aggression-modifying effects primarily by acting directly or indirectly on the brain mechanisms that generate and control aggressive behaviour. An understanding of the influences of alcohol on aggression thus requires knowledge of both the effects of alcohol on the brain and the relationships between brain and behaviour. Unfortunately, both are poorly understood, and very few studies have actually been designed to directly relate alcohol-induced changes in the nervous system to aggression. Even where alcohol-induced changes in brain function can be determined and correlated with behavioural changes, demonstration of causal relationships is impossible. Additional problems are posed by the fact that different 'types' of aggression probably involve different brain mechanisms. Subtle differences in aggression-testing methodology and alcohol administration may yield different results even when the same strain or species of animal is used. These limitations mean that interpretation of data is often difficult, and results from different laboratories often conflict. It seems likely, however, that as more information is gained, the relationships between alcohol, aggression, and the nervous system will become much clearer. This section attempts to assess our present state of knowledge of the effects of alcohol on the nervous system, relating this where possible to aggressive behaviour. Animal studies have usually provided the most detailed information but clinical experiments will be mentioned where relevant.

Cellular Mechanisms of Alcohol Action

Neuropharmacology of Alcohol. The mammalian brain contains many millions of nerve cells. Indeed, the human brain contains some 10^{10} neurons and a much larger number of non-nervous glial cells. These enormous numbers might be expected to make studies at the cellular level of limited value for understanding the neural control of behaviour. While it may be impossible to explain the functions of the integrated nervous system in terms of the known functions of single neurons, nevertheless knowledge of basic nerve mechanisms provides an essential foundation for more general studies. Knowledge of the mechanisms by which alcohol changes the functioning of individual nerve cells is fundamental to any explanation of acute central nervous effects, and provides a first step towards understanding the problems underlying central nervous tolerance and dependence.

Fortunately, the brain has a number of features which simplify its study. It is *not* a random collection of neurons, but is divided into discrete groups of nerve cells (nuclei) which have more-or-less specific behavioural functions and which communicate with each other along specific pathways (tracts). Information is passed along neurons in the tracts in the form of nerve impulses. Interactions between neurons occur at specialised junctions (synapses) where impulses release chemicals (neurotransmitters) from the neuron which interact with receptor molecules on neighbouring (postsynaptic) cells to open or close particular ion channels. Depending on the inorganic ions involved, and the prevailing electrochemical forces, the postsynaptic neurons will tend to be either excited or inhibited. Thirty or more chemicals are thought to act as neurotransmitters, and many more may exist. They may also be released over relatively wide areas of the brain to modulate the activity of large populations of neurons. Indeed, chemical interactions in the brain are much more complex than painted by the classical picture of specific point-to-point, one-way synaptic contacts.

Besides the anatomical orderliness, another feature which has greatly simplified study of brain function is that neurons in particular nuclei and tracts tend to behave similarly and to contain and release the same transmitter. Many psychoactive drugs more-or-less specifically affect a particular transmitter system — for example, certain anti-depressants are thought to act by potentiating transmission at particular synapses that utilise noradrenaline as a transmitter.[1] Many anti-psychotic drugs appear to act by attaching to certain dopamine receptors and blocking them, thus preventing dopamine released at the synapse from activating postsynaptic cells.[1] Tranquillising drugs, such as benzodiazepines (e.g. 'Valium') appear to modify the effects of the transmitter γ-aminobutyric acid.[1] Specificity is far from complete, but the drugs have particular targets in the brain such as receptor sites for neurotransmitters. Neurons lacking these targets will be relatively unaffected (at least directly) except perhaps at very high concentrations.

Alcohol differs, however, from the above type of drug in having no special target (a property shared with certain other depressant drugs such as barbiturates and volatile anaesthetics). Alcohol exerts *non-specific* effects on cell membranes. The cell membrane consists of a lipid bilayer with phosphate and other polar groups directed towards the outer and inner surfaces, and non-polar hydrocarbon chains of fatty acids directed towards the central part of the membrane (Figure 2.1).

Figure 2.1: Schematic Diagram Showing the Organisation of Molecules in the Nerve Cell Membrane

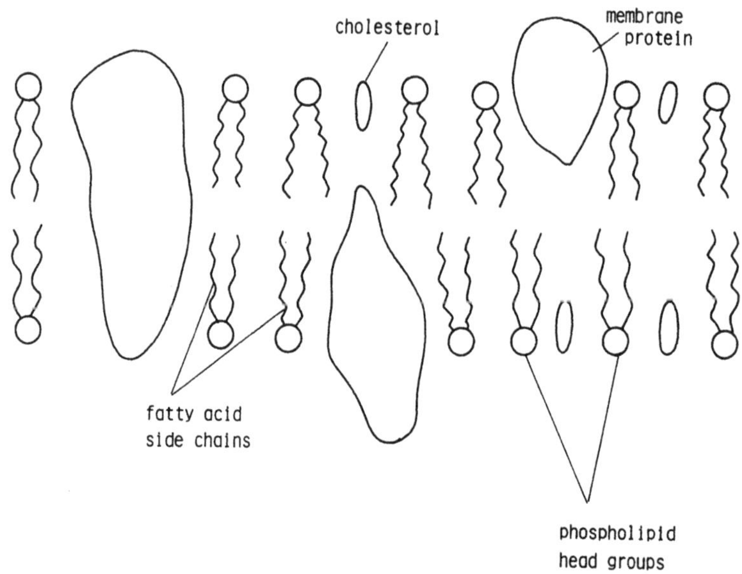

Note: There is a double layer of phospholipids and cholesterol with proteins 'floating' on the surfaces or traversing the entire bilayer (about 10^{-8}m thick). Alcohol enters the lipid portion of the membrane and disrupts its structure which in turn disrupts the proteins that are important for many aspects of neural activity. Chronic intake leads to changes in the lipid composition of the membrane which make it resistant to alcohol (tolerance). On cessation of heavy drinking it takes time for the normal membrane composition to re-establish, and this is at least partly responsible for withdrawal effects which may include episodes of aggression.

Functionally important proteins are situated on the surfaces of the bilayer, some traversing the entire membrane. Proteins are involved in most aspects of neuronal activity, for example providing channels for flow of ions and receptors for neurotransmitters. Unlike most specific drugs such as those mentioned earlier which directly influence particular targets, alcohol appears to exert its main effects indirectly by dissolving in the lipid bilayer and expanding and fluidising the membrane. Normally the lipid molecules are held in a structured arrangement by inter-molecular forces between the lipid molecules themselves, and between them and the proteins. Insertion of alcohol molecules into the lipid of the membrane disrupts its structure and produces a more random and mobile (fluid) arrangement. This alteration in the lipid environment of a protein may alter its functioning. The lipids are not homogeneous and are not all affected to the same extent; thus the effect on a protein will depend on its precise lipid environment. The action of a protein may be increased in one neuron, but the same substance in a different neuron having a different lipid environment, may be totally unaffected or altered in the opposite direction. More direct effects on proteins are also possible, such as interactions with hydrophobic regions of the molecule, but there appears to be no specific receptor site.[2]

There are two major consequences of the above observations. First, it is impossible to predict the effect of alcohol on most neuronal properties. Alcohol can, for example, increase or decrease: (a) the synthesis, storage, release and inactivation of central neurotransmitter substances; (b) resting membrane potential and resistance; (c) neuronal excitability; and (d) postsynaptic receptor sensitivity; in each case only certain cells are affected and different concentrations of alcohol may have opposite effects (Figure 2.2). An enormously diverse range of unpredictable actions is possible, depending on the nature of the lipid environment of the altered process and its sensitivity to membrane perturbations.

In contrast to drugs with specific targets, one cannot directly reverse the neurophysiological effects of alcohol. For example, morphine-like substances have specific receptors and highly localised sites of action, and a heroin overdose can be treated with drugs that specifically block the receptor and stop the heroin action. No single drug can antagonise alcohol's multitude of effects, although individual aspects may be indirectly antagonised

Figure 2.2: Schematic Diagram Showing the Major Features of Nerve Cells

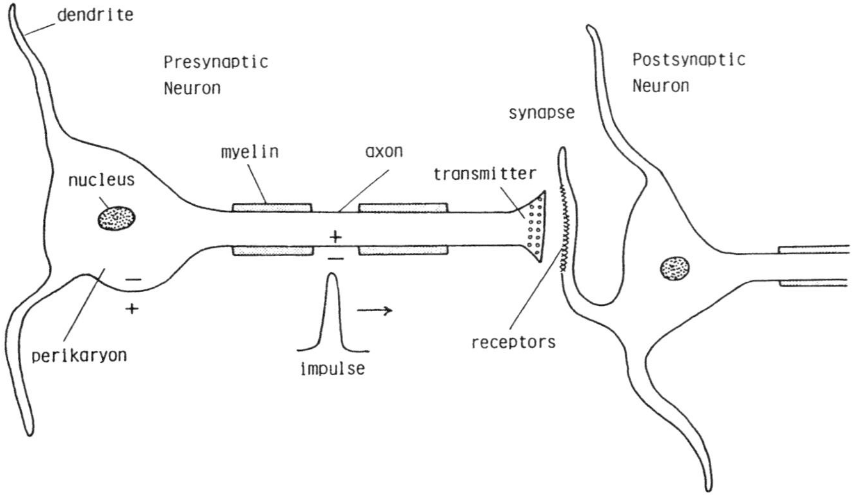

Note: Impulses (brief reversals of the membrane potential) are conducted along the axon to the terminal where they cause release of a neurotransmitter substance on to receptors on the postsynaptic neuron. Transmitter-receptor binding causes opening of ion channels in the membrane, and the resulting current flow tends either to excite or inhibit the postsynaptic neuron. Activity depends on unequal concentrations of individual ions on either side of the nerve membrane, and such concentration gradients are maintained by energy-requiring 'pumps' which transport ions across the membrane. Many properties of nerve cells are influenced by alcohol in a complex manner. Different cells react in opposite ways to alcohol, high concentrations often reverse the effects of low concentrations, and the picture is further complicated by indirect effects *via* other neurons. Chronic exposure to ethanol may result in some recovery of normal function or the production of compensatory changes elsewhere (tolerance). Excessively heavy drinking produces structural changes, e.g. lesions in the myelin (which insulates axons and ensures rapid impulse conduction) and changes in the morphology of dendrites (input regions of the cell which are important integrating sites). Marked increases in cell death occur in certain areas and gross structural brain damage is evident.

and reversed. The best chance for a complete alcohol antagonist (amethystic agent) would probably be a drug that could rapidly inactivate alcohol by 'binding' to it or rapidly converting it to an inactive metabolite.[3]

All membrane-dependent processes (such as active transport systems, hormonal interaction, the immune response and the cell-cell recognition process) may be affected by alcohol to some extent.[4] Wide variations in sensitivity occur, however, so that particular cells may show gross impairment of function while others show no measurable changes. Different regions of a cell may show marked variation in sensitivity also, and it is generally accepted that synaptic mechanisms are more susceptible to alcohol than, for example, the generation of action potentials. Changes at synapses appear to underlie most of the central effects of alcohol except perhaps at near-lethal doses. Although this is a good general rule, and most attention has been focused on synaptic mechanisms, it would be unwise to disregard other (perhaps subtle) changes in neuronal function such as pattern of firing.[5]

Neurophysiological Effects of Alcohol. Most of our knowledge of the cellular effects of alcohol has been obtained from invertebrates or from vertebrate neurons lying outside the central nervous system (CNS). It is usually much easier to apply high-resolution techniques to such systems, and data can be interpreted more reliably. Caution is obviously required in attempting to extrapolate such results to the mammalian brain, but it appears that the main differences between, for example, invertebrate and vertebrate nervous systems are in the number and precise connectivity of neurons and not in individual cell properties. The basic principles of generation of resting membrane potential, impulse conduction and all the aspects of synaptic transmission appear remarkably similar, and in the main, the same neurotransmitters are used. Although experiments on invertebrates and the peripheral systems of vertebrates do not provide a substitute for looking directly at effects on the mammalian CNS they do help in the interpretation of the usually much more complex data obtained from the mammalian brain. The introduction of more sophisticated techniques will make it possible to probe single-neuron properties in the brain more directly.

Alcohol generally has a biphasic action on neuronal excitability;[6,7] low concentrations tend to increase excitability (i.e. they produce a lower stimulus threshold) whilst high concentrations transiently increase and then progressively reduce excitability (and spike amplitude), leading eventually to a complete block of impulse conduction. The stimulant and depressant concentrations of alcohol vary widely in different excitable structures, but complete block generally occurs only at alcohol concentrations that are higher than can be tolerated *in vivo*. It is difficult to distinguish in the CNS between direct and indirect effects of systemically administered alcohol on the excitability of individual neurons. Direct microinjection of alcohol via a micropipette is either ineffective, or increases or decreases the firing rate of individual neurons in the mammalian cortex [8] and hypothalamus.[9] Changes in firing pattern also may occur, such as the production of bursts of neuronal activity.[5,10] This may reflect the intermediate effects of alcohol between depression and activation.[10]

The effects on excitability and conduction have been regarded by some investigators as the principal mechanism by which alcohol produces intoxication. Others have favoured a wholly synaptic mechanism (see ref. 11 for discussion of these arguments). Excitatory synapses are certainly sensitive to and are often depressed by alcohol.[12] It has been generally accepted that the stimulant effects of alcohol are due to disinhibition[13] (i.e. alcohol produces excitation indirectly by specifically reducing inhibitory inputs). The effects of alcohol on synaptic transmission are not, however, always depressant, as alcohol directly potentiates excitatory transmission in cat spinal cord[14] and at the neuromuscular junction in amphibia and mammals.[15,16] Of course, if pathways excited by alcohol themselves inhibit other neurons, the end result could still be one of depression. Alcohol can, however, directly potentiate inhibition.[17]

Alcohol may thus increase or decrease both excitatory and inhibitory transmission; there is no apparent distinction between the two. Some of the effects on transmission may be subtle and difficult to identify, such as the alcohol-increased rate of decay of post-tetanic potentiation (PTP) at the mammalian neuromuscular junction[18] and in the nervous system of the marine mollusc *Aplysia*.[19] PTP is the increased efficacy of synaptic transmission which occurs after repetitive (tetanic) stimulation at certain synapses, and results from increased transmitter release. In *Aplysia* the effect on PTP decay is selective since there is no effect on a single excitatory postsynaptic potential, on synaptic depression and facilitation or on the maximum amplitude of PTP.[19] In conclusion, evidence is increasing that alcohol exerts many of its central nervous effects by *specific* modulation of synaptic transmission rather than by general depression of membrane responsiveness.

Effects of Alcohol on Brain Regions Associated with Aggression

Alcohol appears likely to affect all brain regions, but it would seem appropriate to focus, at least initially, on those areas most intimately concerned with the expression of aggressive behaviour. One way to identify such areas is by brain stimulation. The first of such studies were made by Hess,[20] who developed the chronic brain electrode technique to allow stimulation of unanaesthetised animals while they moved freely. Initial studies described and categorised both skeletal and autonomic reactions, and provided a wealth of important data, but the experiments were limited by failure to provide an appropriate target such as a conspecific or prey animal to react to. The subsequent utilisation of animate targets and the recording of attack episodes have significantly advanced the understanding of the brain mechanisms for aggression.

Stimulation of many different brain sites will elicit aggressive behaviour. Although historically the hypothalamus was the most important structure, recent data seem to reduce its importance. Fibres passing through the structure have been assigned many of the functions previously ascribed to hypothalamic cells and 'centres' themselves.[21] Depending on the precise stimulation area, the resulting behaviour may be primarily one of defence (defensive attack), offence or predatory aggression. The areas involved in defence are the best mapped, and involve the amygdala and parts of the brain stem central grey.[21]

MacDonnell and Ehmer[22] and MacDonnell and Fessock[23] studied the effects of alcohol on stimulus-induced attack by a cat on an anaesthetised rat. The duration of the attack is determined by the duration of brain stimulation, and its intensity is easily controlled by manipulating stimulus intensity. The behaviour is precisely coordinated and is accompanied by a minimum of sympathetic display, unlike affective defence which may be accompanied by snarling, screeching, slashing and spitting. The former response was originally described as a 'quiet biting attack'.[24] Alcohol has been found to increase attack latency with increasing dose. Alcohol also causes problems of head orientation and difficulties in jaw opening. The cat often sweeps its muzzle back and forth over the target but the reflexive opening of the jaws (in response to tactile stimulation of certain perioral zones) is either greatly delayed or completely absent. The force of biting is, however, increased by alcohol. In electrophysiological experiments doses of alcohol as low as 0.17g/kg depressed the evoked response of the pool of trigeminal motoneurons activated by stimulation of pathways from the basal ganglia.[23]

MacDonnell, Fessock and Brown[25] have also studied the effects of alcohol on affective defence elicited by stimulation of the hypothalamic ventromedial nucleus, and the modulatory effects of stimulating the amygdala. A low alcohol dose (0.37g/kg) produced hyperexcitability (as evidenced for example by a shorter hissing latency) while a moderate dose (1.5g/kg) produced initial hyperexcitability, then a depression followed by rebound hyperexcitability and a return to normal. Small amounts of alcohol facilitated overt vocal behaviour characteristic of affective defence, and increased the amplitudes of evoked potentials in the hypothalamic ventromedial nucleus in response to stimulation of amygdaloid structures having known facilitative influences on affective defence. Moderate doses of alcohol had the opposite effect on the latter phenomenon and, during recovery, there was a rebound hyperexcitability. These experiments provide a possibly direct neural correlate of the biphasic actions of alcohol on aggressive behaviour that have been described in many animals (see Chapter 4). The relevance of these stimulation studies to hostile behaviour in normal (unstimulated) confrontations with other cats is unknown, but this type of experiment seems an excellent approach to the study of alcohol and aggression, particularly since it has been coupled with neurochemical manipulations (see below).

Johannson[26] has confirmed that alcohol has an excitatory effect on affective defence at low doses in intact, unstimulated cats, but depresses behaviour at high concentrations. Defence behaviour was elicited here not by electrical stimulation but by exposure to a threatening cat. Threat was ingeniously controlled and standardised in the stimulus animal by electrical brain stimulation.

Neural substrates of aggression have also been studied by destroying discrete brain areas, but the results have been less than conclusive.[21] Localised lesions have provided useful information, but the study of the roles played by specific brain regions on the release of aggressive behaviour is now regarded as over-simplistic;[27] the diversity of the brain mechanisms involved in aggressive behaviour shows that there is no single 'aggression centre' in the brain.[28] Besides the neural structures that elicit or modulate aggressive behaviour more-or-less independently of the environment, it is also necessary to study the sensory and motor systems which are biased so that the organism acts aggressively in certain specific ways depending on the presence of an appropriate stimulus.[27] The response of a cat stimulated in the lateral hypothalamus will be different in the presence of a rat or when confronting a dominant or submissive partner. The experimental situation greatly influences and may even reverse the effects of brain stimulation.[29] Similar problems exist with ablation studies; bilateral lesions of specific septal nuclei in a number of species induces 'irritable aggression' and yet decreases dominance and competitive aggression.[30]

It is possible that electrical stimulation of some of the brain sites that elicit or modulate aggressive behaviour may alter the biasing of common sensorimotor mechanisms. Electrical stimulation has the disadvantage that both nearby cell bodies (i.e. parts of the cell with important integrative capabilities) and axons passing through the area (i.e. simple conducting parts of the cell) are excited by the stimulating current. Recently, however, aggressive behaviour has been elicited by microinjection of excitatory amino acids which specifically stimulate cell bodies.[27] This should assist one in identifying the pathways and sensorimotor mechanisms which mediate the behavioural consequences of excitation of these neurons.

In conclusion, it may be said that alcohol may act on one or more of the following: (i) brain mechanisms directly associated with the generation of aggressive behaviour; (ii) brain mechanisms that specifically facilitate or inhibit the activity of a given motivational system, thus increasing or reducing the tendency to emit the motivated behaviour in response to the relevant stimuli; and (iii) the way in which the brain perceives an individually determined relationship to a given situation, and on the way it anticipates, on the basis of its prior experience, a method to cope with it by using particular components of its behavioural repertoire.[28]

This involves study of a number of interacting processes that do not appear to be specifically related to a particular behavioural pattern. The operations involved in the processing of sensory input occur against the background of the individual's overall excitability and emotional reactivity. Furthermore, the actual significance and consequently the actual behavioural effects of a given sensory input clearly depend on the individual's prior experience.[28] Less specific brain activity could underlie the variability of alcohol-induced effects which may heavily depend on experiential variables.

Chronic Effects of Alcohol: Development of Tolerance and Dependence

Chronic (repeated) administration of alcohol leads to tolerance, where more drug is required to produce the same behavioural and physiological effects. Conversely, a subject is able to function almost normally after doses of alcohol that previously produced impairment. This is partly the result of an enhanced ability to metabolise alcohol[31] but mainly due to an adaptive process of the nervous system — a degree of tolerance can occur within minutes or hours after a single dose of alcohol and is known as 'acute tolerance'.[32] Full tolerance in mice takes about three days to develop, and has been shown to occur at the level of the synaptic membrane which becomes resistant to the fluidising (i.e. disruptive) effects of alcohol.

A number of membrane changes have been observed in response to chronic alcohol treatment, such as reduced proportions of polyunsaturated fatty acids in phospholipids of the synaptic membrane.[33] The problem now is to determine which membrane changes contribute to the development of alcohol tolerance and in what way. The change in fatty-acid composition would be expected to increase rigidity of the membrane and diminish its susceptibility to fluidisation by alcohol, but many other changes occur whose significance is unknown. An additional point to bear in mind is that the membrane composition is in a dynamic state, with individual components continually 'turning over' (i.e. being broken down and then reformed). It is possible that a change in turnover in certain membrane constituents may contribute to the production of tolerance even though their overall composition remains the same.[33]

The membrane thus becomes adapted to function in the presence of alcohol but not in its absence (i.e. there is a state of alcohol dependence), and this may be the cause of withdrawal symptoms which occur on cessation of drinking until the membrane readjusts to the alcohol-free condition. The situation is actually more complicated than this,[34,35] and different types of adaptive changes may be involved. For example, a prolonged reduction in transmitter release (which may occur in chronic alcoholics) causes the postsynaptic membrane to become much more sensitive to the transmitter, tending to return transmission to normal. Tolerance thus probably depends on a number of different mechanisms.

Many changes in brain chemistry and physiology have been associated with chronic alcohol administration, but few attempts have been made to relate these to altered aggressive behaviour. As withdrawal from alcohol is well known to produce an excited state with aggressive episodes,[36] this would seem a fruitful area for further research.

Alcohol and Brain Damage

It seems likely that in most cases of acute intoxication there is no irreversible damage to the brain, and this organ's functions quickly recover. Brain damage is, however, a feature of the chronic alcoholic, and should therefore be considered as a possible mechanism for altering the propensity for aggressive behaviour. Malnutrition (especially thiamine deficiency) has often been claimed to be a major cause of severe CNS impairment in chronic alcoholics, but controlled studies demonstrate that direct neurotoxic effects of alcohol are more important.[37] Animal experiments are particularly valuable in this respect because in humans there are many other coexisting variables such as nutrition, environment, aging, heredity, exposure to other toxic agents or head trauma.[37] These toxic actions probably reflect a generalised cell-damaging effect of alcohol, though certain brain areas seem particularly susceptible. Five months of chronic alcohol intake by rodents has been shown to result in significant neuronal loss in the hippocampus, dentate gyrus and cerebellum. Alterations were also found in the morphology of dendrites (input regions of nerve cells), which represent either an early phase of a progressive degenerative reaction terminating in neuronal death or a parallel neuropathological alteration.[37] There were, however, no detectable alterations in the medial thalamus or striatum.[37] The non-invasive technique of computerised axial tomography (a special computer-assisted X-ray technique) has confirmed a high incidence of cerebral atrophy in even quite young alcoholics.[38]

The mechanism of neurotoxic action of alcohol is unknown; the drug could be directly toxic or exert its effects indirectly, for example by the reduction of cerebral blood flow to specific brain regions.[39] Chronic alcohol does not, however, appear to damage the blood brain barrier which regulates the flow of substances into and out of the brain.[40,41]

The neuropathological and behavioural changes associated with chronic alcoholism in man are similar to those due to ageing, and it has been suggested that chronic alcoholism may accelerate the aging process.[42] Attempts have been made to correlate the damaged regions with the impaired memory that occurs in many chronic alcoholics. Similarly, the collection of quantitative behavioural and neurohistological data on the same set of animals following prolonged alcohol consumption should help to clarify the relationship between the aggressive and regional neuropathological *sequelae* of alcohol abuse.

It is possible that some of the intoxicating and toxic effects of alcohol are caused by its metabolites rather than by alcohol itself (see Chapter 6). Acetaldehyde has been shown to be responsible for the alcohol intolerance shown by most Orientals, whereby small amounts of alcohol may cause symptoms such as nausea, headache, tachycardia, weakness and facial flushing.[43] The drug Disulfiram is sometimes administered to chronic alcoholics to discourage drinking; acetaldehyde synthesis from alcohol is not affected but its breakdown is prevented, and unpleasant symptoms are produced by even small amounts of alcohol. Besides a possible direct cffect of acetaldehyde on nervous tissue, interest has recently focused on substances which are formed by the reaction of acetaldehyde with the neurotransmitters dopamine and noradrenaline. Some of these substances (tetrahydroisoquinolines or TIQs) have been detected in the brain of rodents following chronic administration of alcohol[44] and in urine of patients suffering from Parkinson's disease who drink alcohol while receiving l-DOPA therapy (aimed to increase dopamine levels).[45] TIQs have various pharmacological properties and appear to act as false transmitters,[46] i.e. they displace the natural transmitter but show only weak receptor activation. Few behavioural studies have been made, but rats given chronic intraventricular injections of TIQs vastly increase alcohol intake when given a choice between water and dilute alcohol solutions. Although TIQs are quickly inactivated, the effect on alcohol preference lasts for months, suggesting that they may act as neurotoxins.[44]

TIQs are related to highly addictive opiate drugs (e.g. morphine and heroin), and speculations rage that they could be involved in alcohol addiction. Many other substances are formed from the reactions of acetaldehyde, and it will be interesting to see whether any of the behavioural effects of chronic alcohol consumption prove to be mediated by these substances.

Alcohol and Neurotransmitters

Major advances have been made in elucidating the neurochemical bases of behaviour by the identification of biochemically specific pathways in the brain. This makes it possible to modify selected brain areas with (more-or-less) specific transmitter-modifying drugs administered by injection or orally (i.e. without having to inject directly into the appropriate brain areas). These agents modify effects of specific neurotransmitters by acting on their synthesis, storage, release, activation of receptors, or inactivation. If a particular transmitter pathway is involved in the neural circuitry underlying a particular form of aggressive behaviour, then the drug-induced modifications are likely to alter the behaviour. There has been a tendency to relate specific types of behaviour to single brain chemicals, but this is obviously an over-simplification since many different neurotransmitters are usually involved. Nevertheless, modification of some transmitters may produce much greater effects than others. As a variety of transmitter systems have been implicated in the modulation of aggressive behaviour and all have been found to be modified by alcohol, it is difficult to identify the specific systems responsible for alcohol-induced changes in behaviour. For example, isolation-induced aggression is generally inhibited by drugs that increase noradrenergic transmission. Paradoxically, several agents that reduce noradrenergic transmission also inhibit isolation-induced aggression.[47] The action of alcohol on neurotransmitters is also confusing, and apparently contradictory results abound for all the transmitter systems studied in detail. For example, alcohol causes an initial increase of synthesis and release of neural noradrenaline.[48] Experiments on brain slices or synaptosomes (isolated fragments of synaptic terminals) *in vitro,* however, show that alcohol reduces release,[49] and iontophoresis experiments show that noradrenaline receptors have a reduced sensitivity after alcohol administration.[8] Littleton[50] suggests that the paradox may be resolved by supposing that the initial, apparently stimulatory effect of alcohol on central noradrenaline in the intact animal is an indirect effect, mediated by the non-specific stress involved in administration of large, acute doses of alcohol. The likely direct effect of alcohol on noradrenergic terminals seems to be an inhibition of transmitter release which accompanies a reduction in receptor sensitivity and hence reduced functional activity.[50]

Experiments on the effects of alcohol on neurotransmitters unfortunately tend to be carried out separately (and by different workers) from experiments on the relationship between neurotransmitters and aggression. The equivocal nature of much of the data, and the fact that slight differences in methodology yield different results, makes it essential to try to determine relationships directly. MacDonnell, Fessock and Brown[51] studied the effect of alcohol on brain-stimulated predatory attack and affective defence in cats while reducing brain serotonin levels with p-chlorophenylalanine or injecting serotonin into selected brain areas. They concluded that: (i) low doses of alcohol block serotonin-modulated hypothalamic events regulating the expression of affective defence; (ii) moderate doses of alcohol enhance such serotonin-modulated events; and (iii) during the later phases of recovery from moderate alcohol doses (during rebound hyperexcitability), another period of blocking of serotonin-modulated events might be expected. The data did not however, indicate any particular mechanism, and it was concluded that almost any hypothetical position could find support.[51] The situation remains much the same today.

In conclusion, it appears that each type of 'aggression' has its own characteristic multi-transmitter profile. As transmitters probably act in a balanced manner, and alcohol alters this balance, aggression is changed. Unfortunately, most experimental data provide no clear picture. For example, it is difficult to implicate particular neurotransmitter systems in the effects of alcohol because they are all to some extent directly or indirectly affected by the drug. Also the results of experiments are often inconsistent, e.g. the concentration of the neurotransmitter γ-aminobutyric acid (GABA) has been found to be increased, unchanged, or decreased by alcohol by various workers.[11] Indeed Sytinsky, Guzikov, Gomanko, Eremin and Konovalova[52] reported that low doses of alcohol slightly increased GABA levels in the cerebellum and cerebral hemispheres, larger doses decreased it, and lethal doses produced a sharp increase. Such multi-phasic effects may explain some of the apparent contradictions in the literature. Pohorecky and Jaffe[48] found that 1g/kg alcohol reduced noradrenaline metabolites 30 min later whereas the reverse was the case at 60 min. The presence of such biphasic effects means that it is essential in comparative studies to consider the dose of alcohol and time of experimental tests among other things.

It should further be noted that some of alcohol's central nervous effects may depend on whether or not the liver is damaged. The liver is particularly susceptible to alcohol, possibly because of the high concentration of acetaldehyde found in this tissue. The liver has been suggested to play a role in the central neurotransmitter changes which accompany acute and chronic alcohol administration.[50] Alcohol acts on the liver to alter the levels of certain transmitter precursors in plasma (i.e. inactive substances which are converted to active transmitters in the brain) and this may influence transmitter metabolism in the brain. An indirect effect of alcohol on neurotransmitters via alteration of hepatic functioning may thus be very important.

Alcohol and Endocrinology

The word 'endocrinology' is derived from the Greek roots: *endon* (within), *krinein* (to separate) and *logos* (to study). This subject principally relates to the study of the endocrine or ductless glands which secrete their product directly into the bloodstream. Such glands are found throughout the Metazoa, but reach their highest degree of sophistication in the vertebrates. The products of the endocrine glands are known as *hormones* (from the Greek *hormon* to excite) and the glands may be classed as *effector organs* i.e. structures that bring about specific responses to stimuli (cf sensory organs that receive stimuli). An indication of their basic action is provided in Figure 2.3.

The endocrine glands influence homeostasis which in its widest sense is the coordinated physiological processes which maintain the constancy of the organism's internal environment. Homeostasis does not imply a lack of change, as the 'steady state' which the complex regulatory mechanisms maintain may shift from time to time, but throughout changes, factors remain under more-or-less close control. These mechanisms which include behavioural change are, of course, essential for the continued existence of organisms living in fluctuating environments.

Figure 2.3: Diagrammatic Representation of a Chain of Endocrine Events

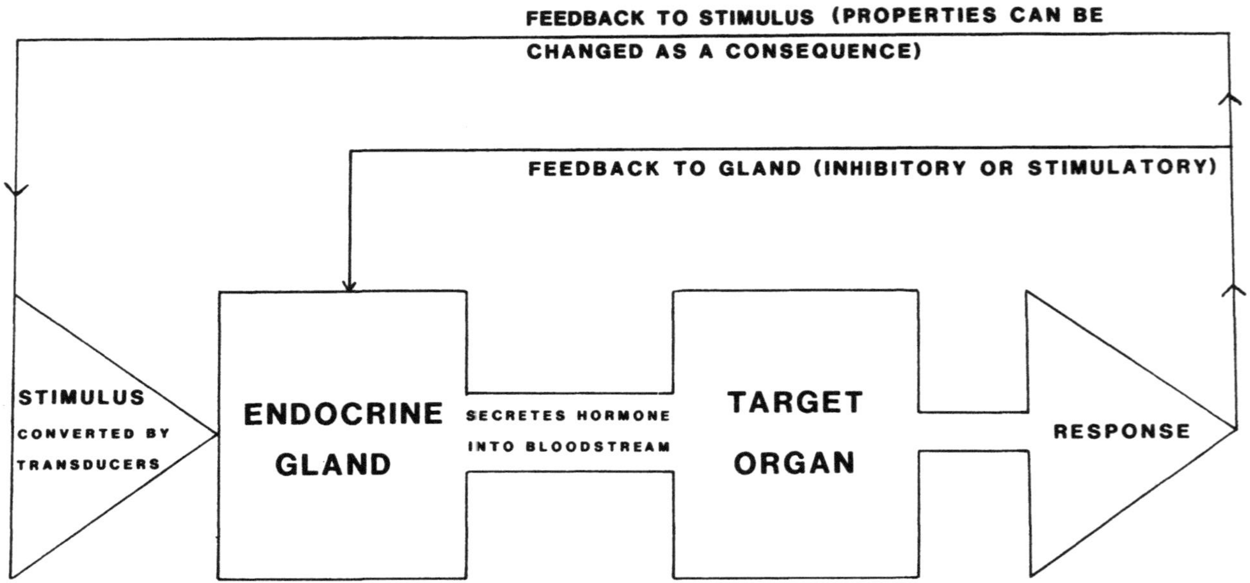

Note: the stimulus can be received direct, via a sense organ or via one or more preceeding glands. The term 'transducer' is used as the form of the stimulus is generally converted into another form of energy. The coupling between receptor (whether 'direct' as in neuroendocrine structures or perhaps by occupying binding sites) and the endocrine gland's hormone synthesis/release machinery differs between different glands and with respect to particular activators. The hormonal action on target organ cells follows an analogous pattern. In many cases the cellular mediation of hormone effects depends on unknown components as is the case in the CNS. The response is often related to the production of hormone in a negative feedback relationship (as in an aquarium thermostat), but other relationships including positive feedback may be apparent.

Hormones, according to Bayliss and Starling[53] are (a) identifiable chemical secretions of endocrine glands; and are (b) transported to their site(s) of action in the bloodstream. Currently, however, the division of information-carrying molecules into 'hormones' and 'assorted chemical messengers' seems distinctly arbitrary. What, for example, is the status of active factors that derive from non-glandular cells and can have both local and distant targets (e.g. histamine and prostaglandins)?

The major endocrine structures in a rat and a man are shown in Figure 2.4. The constancy of these structures in very diverse organisms is remarkable.

Actions and Hormones

It seems useful to provide initially a synopsis of the major secretions of specific endocrine glands in mammals and to relate this to basic actions on principal target tissues (see Table 2.2). The point to be remembered is that the endocrine system, like the brain, is a highly integrated web of dynamic relationships, and that *any* deformation of that system (such as might be induced by alcohol ingestion) is likely to have repercussions throughout the entire body. It is consequently hardly remarkable that it is impossible to identify a single physiological consequence of ethanol that one can relate to a behavioural change.

Hormones and Alcohol

The involvement of ethanol in endocrine changes has been studied in detail often because the hormonal variation has been thought to account for altered behavioural effects such as in the case of aggressiveness. It should be noted, however, that hormones do *not* cause behaviour in the simple sense[54] and that behaviour may modulate hormones as well as vice versa. One must also reiterate that different 'kinds' of aggression are influenced to differing degrees by particular hormonal systems. Although ethanol produces many biochemical perturbations with a complex patterning, it seems worth examining the recorded effects in animals and man system by system.

Neurally Active Peptides. Repeated claims have been made about the association between ethanol administration and endogenous opioids and other neurally active peptides. For example, Luttinger, Nemeroff, Mason, Frye, Breese and Prange[55] have noted that

Figure 2.4: Simplified Representation of the Position of Some of the Major Endocrine Glands Within the Bodies of Man and the Rat

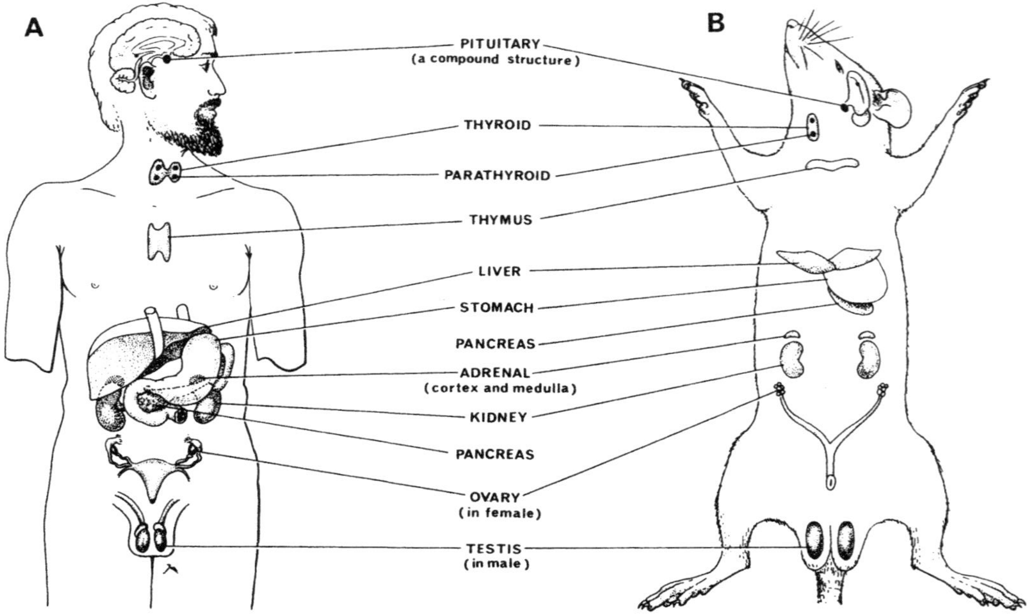

Note: The locations of endocrine glands are similar in all mammalian species (reproduced from Brain, P.F. in *Chemical Influences on Behaviour* (eds K. Brown and S.J. Cooper), Academic Press: London, 1979).

Table 2.2: Synopsis of the Putative Endocrine Glands, Their Secretions and Particular Functions in Mammals

Gland	Secretions	Target tissues/Functions
Nervous system	Hormone-like factors located in the central nervous system/peripheral nervous system. (*compounds found in sensory afferents and **those in autonomic efferent axons)	All presumed to have neuromodulator (in some cases neurotransmitter) actions
	Thyrotropin-releasing hormone	Thyrotrophs of anterior pituitary — releases thyroid stimulating hormone
	Luteinizing hormone-releasing factor	Gonadotrophs of anterior pituitary — releases luteinizing hormone and (perhaps) follicle stimulating hormone
	Somatostatin	Somatotrophs of anterior pituitary — inhibits growth hormone release
	Melanocyte-stimulating hormone-release-inhibiting factor	Cells of pars intermedia — inhibits release of melanocyte stimulating hormone
	Neurotensins Substance P* Enkephalins ** Bombesin Gastrin	See section on gut endocrines — several of these peptides affect one or more aspect of anterior pituitary hormone release
	Renin-Angiotensin Vasopressin Oxytocin	All these substances directly or indirectly affect anterior pituitary function
	Endorphins B Lipotrophin Melanocyte-stimulating hormone Adrenocorticotrophic hormone	All may affect pituitary and neural functions
Pineal gland	Melatonin (other methoxyindoles) Pinealotypical peptides	Hypothalamus (inhibits release of MSH and gonadotrophins), contracts melanophores (in lower vertebrates)

Table 2.2 continued

Pituitary Adenohypophysis (Pars distalis)	Follicle-stimulating hormone	Stimulates follicular development in the ovary; stimulates gametogenesis in the testes
	Luteinizing hormone, (also called interstitial-cell-stimulating hormone)	Promotes luteinization of the ovary; stimulates Leydig cell function of the testes
	Thyrotrophic hormone	Stimulates thyroid hormone release and synthesis; promotes lipolysis in adipose tissue
	Adrenocorticotrophic hormone	Releases glucocorticoids from adrenocortical tissue; affects various aspects of CNS function
	Growth hormone, (somatotrophic hormone)	Liver; forms somatomedin, which alters tissue metabolism (liver, muscle, adipose tissue); stimulates tissue growth and protein synthesis
	Prolactin (luteotrophic hormone)	Mammary glands, corpus luteum, skin, and so on. Initiates and maintains lactation and maternal behavioural homeostasis. Promotes growth, progesterone secretion, synergism with steroids
Pars intermedia	β-lipotrophin Melanocyte-stimulating hormone	Adipose tissue deposition. Contains sequences of opioid-like peptides (endorphins) functions unclear in mammals, but modulates some behavioural processes
Neurohypophysis	Vasopressin (Argenine or lysine (pig) form)	Kidney; conserves body water (antidiuretic) — modulates learning and memory processes
	Oxytocin	Affects lactation and uterine muscle contraction
Thyroid gland	Thyroxine/Triiodothyronine	Tissue metabolism and differentiation, calorigenic (mammals)
Parathyroid gland	Parathormone	Bone, kidney and gut-hypercalcaemic
Ultimobranchial bodies ('C' cells in mammalian thyroid)	Calcitonin, (also called thyrocalcitonin)	Bone and kidney-hypocalcaemic
Adrenal glands Cortex (interrenals in sharks and rays)	Cortisol, corticosterone cortisone, 1α-hydroxycorticosterone	Liver and muscle; proteins to amino acids, gluconeogenesis. Intestine, skin and gills in teleosts; increased Na^+, K^+-activated ATPase

	Aldosterone	Kidney, sweat and salivary glands, gut, Na^+ and K^+balance
	Sex steroids	Stimulates secondary sexual characteristics etc.
Medulla (chromaffin tissue)	Norepinephrine (noradrenaline) Epinephrine (adrenaline)	Liver, muscle and adipose tissue; glycogenolysis, mobilisation fatty acids, calorigenic, smooth muscle constriction and relaxation
Islets of Langerhans		
α-cells	Glucagon	Liver (glycogenolysis), adipose tissue (fatty acid release)
β-cells	Insulin	Liver, muscle, and adipose tissue; amino acid or protein, glucose to fat and glycogen
δ-cells	Somatostatin	See earlier
Gonads		
Ovary		
Graafian follicle	Oestrogens	Female sex organs and characters (mammary glands, brain)
Corpus luteum	Progestins	Uterus, mammary glands and brain
Testis		
Interstitial tissue (Leydig cells)	Androgens	Male sex organs and characters sperm maturation, brain
Sertoli cells (?)	Androgens	Sperm maturation
Placenta (pregnant eutherian mammals)	Oestrogens Progesterone	Uterus, mammary glands, fetus
	Chorionic gonadotrophin	Stimulates persistence of the corpus luteum
	Placental lactogen, (somatomammotrophin)	Mammary glands
Gut Stomach (pyloric mucosa)	Gastrin	Stomach; stimulates secretion of gastric juices
Duodenum (mucosa)	Enterogastrone (?)	Inhibits secretion of gastric juices, from stomach
	Secretin	Exocrine pancreas: stimulation of pancreatic juices Induces behavioural satiety: stimulates pancreatic secretion

Table 2.2 continued

		Exocrine pancreas and gall bladder; enzyme secretion and release of bile
	Glucagon	See Islets of langerhans
Kidney		
Tubular cells	1,25-dihydroxy-cholecalciferol	Bone and intestine; resorption of calcium
Juxtaglomerular cells	Renin	Plasma α globulin; angiotensin, stimulates adrenal cortex and smooth muscle
	Epithelial growth factor	Skin growth
	Erythropoietin	Red blood cell production

neurotensin, β-endorphin and bombesin all increase the duration of ethanol-induced sleep, and that the first two mentioned compounds alter the hypothermia induced by alcohol. Little and Wing[56] have reviewed the pharmacological links between ethanol and the opiates. For example, the endogenous opiate blocker naloxone antagonises (at high doses) some of the effects of ethanol. There is also evidence (based on rather extreme *in vitro* conditions) that ethanol reduces opioid receptor binding (especially δ-receptors) in brain and may also change the release of endorphins and enkephalins. It has also been suggested that TIQs may be implicated in ethanol's effects on central endogenous opiate systems. ACTH and MSH share peptide sequences which are also said to have neural actions.[57] These preparations may antagonise ethanol's effects on sleeping times in animal experiments.[58]

There is also evidence that alcohol changes the secretion of Argenine vasopressin, and is associated with alterations in diuresis. The effects, however, are variable and difficult to evaluate (reviewed in ref. 59).

Alcohol and Pineal Hormones. There have also been claims[60] that the pineal hormone melatonin may enhance the self-administration of ethanol by laboratory rodents. Such self-administration is also influenced by the animal's light/dark cycle.

Alcohol and Thyroid Function. Thyroid hormones change voluntary alcohol consumption of animals and modify the metabolism and metabolic effects of alcohol (reviewed in ref. 59). Some (but not all) studies suggest that alcoholics are often hypothyroid. Although alcoholics show significantly decreased levels of thyroid hormones and non-significant increases in TSH, such changes may be secondary consequences of liver damage, a condition known to affect metabolism of thyroid hormones.[61] Acute experiments with alcohol do not suggest that this drug significantly alters thyroid hormones or TSH concentrations.[62]

Alcohol and Parathyroid Function. Single or repeated (every 0.5hrs for 2 hrs) doses of ethanol produce lowered blood calcium levels associated with elevated blood magnesium titres in rats.[63] Although it was claimed that this effect is due to impaired parathyroid hormone secretion, Shah, Bowser, Hargis, Wongsurawat, Banerjee, Henderson and Williams[64] were unable to demonstrate any such action. Indeed, augmented parathyroid hormones do not correct the reduced calcium level.

Alcohol and Carbohydrate Metabolism. Ethanol alters carbohydrate metabolism, producing complex disturbances of plasma levels of glucose and changes in sensitivity to insulin in laboratory animals[65] and man.[66] The basic change is that alcohol increases glucose-induced insulin secretion and may consequently cause reactive hypoglycaemia (low blood-sugar levels). It does not seem to be the case, however, that alcohol-induced hypoglycaemia in fasted subjects is a consequence of inappropriate insulin release.[59] Alcohol increases the secretion of glucagon in some animals (rats, pig and man) which may contribute to the depletion of liver carbohydrate stores seen during alcohol intoxication. It has also been claimed on the basis of animal studies, that diabetogenic disturbances predispose individuals to show a preference for alcohol.[67]

Alcohol and Adrenocortical Function. Attempts to associate ethanol intake with altered endocrine function have recently concentrated on the pituitary-adrenocortical axis. There has been a tendency to regard acute and chronic administration of ethanol as a uniformly stressful procedure which produces many pathological changes although it has been noted that it is often claimed that alcohol is drunk to relieve stress.[59] Acute administration (by intragastric or intraperitoneal routes) of ethanol generally increases adrenocortical function in animals.[68] Alcohol modifies the normal circadian rhythm of corticosterone secretion, producing more marked elevations in the normal trough period.[69] Direct evidence has been produced[70] that the increased adrenocortical response in ethanol treated animals is a consequence of augmented ACTH secretion. One should note that ethanol probably impairs both effective food consumption[71] and immune responses,[72] and these may account for some alterations in adrenal function. Indeed Pohorecky and Rizek[73] have suggested that part of the ethanol-mediated increase in corticosterone secretion is a secondary consequence of hypothermia (reduced body temperature). They also found that alcohol impaired motor activity in rats. There may be complex relationships between corticosterone secretion, circadian rhythmicity and experience of ethanol administration, with some phenomena being ameliorated by naloxone administration,[74] suggesting an opioid influencing effect (see p. 27). Some studies[75] suggest that low doses of ethanol may have a stress-relieving effect in rats, reducing the corticosterone response to unavoidable foot shock. As well as alcohol modifying adrenocortical function, there is some evidence that adrenal hormones influence ethanol ingestion. Green[76] has shown that alcohol consumption by mice is significantly depressed by some treatments with hydrocortisone acetate, but is unchanged by deoxycorticosterone acetate. As the former is a glucocorticoid and the latter a mineralocorticoid, she tentatively suggests that glucocorticoids influence alcohol preference in mice.

Evidence has been produced in humans[77] that there is stimulation of the renin-aldosterone axis during ethanol intoxication and hangover. These changes may be due to diuresis, dehydration and increased sympathetic nervous system activation seen following alcohol ingestion.

Alcohol and Adrenomedullary Function. In dogs it has been claimed that the stimulation of insulin by ethanol is a consequence of a reduction of catecholamines.[78] In man, however, the urinary levels of adrenalin and noradrenalin are stable after alcohol administration.[70]

Alcohol and the Pituitary-gonadal Axis. There has been considerable interest in the effects of alcohol on the hormones of the pituitary-gonadal axis. These might be expected to be of particular importance in relation to aggression which is often stereotyped as a male-typical, androgen-dependent activity (the weakness of this view is examined in Brain, Haug and vom Saal[79]). The effects of alcohol on gonadal function have also been reviewed in ref. 59. Alcohol may inhibit the secretion of luteinizing hormone-releasing factor (LHRF) consequently decreasing plasma levels of luteinizing hormone (and hence testosterone in animals). Studies with healthy male and female volunteers in a clinic did *not* confirm that alcohol (in the intoxication, hangover or withdrawal phases) influenced LHRF-induced LH secretion in either gender. The production, metabolism and clearance of testosterone are reduced after ethanol administration (both acute and chronic) in man[80] and a variety of experimental animals.[81] In alcohol addicts intoxication produces falls in plasma levels of testosterone with little change in urinary oestrogens or plasma cortisol.[82] This suppression of testosterone seems due to both direct effects of ethanol on testicular function[83] as well as actions on the pituitary or hypothalamus.[84] Indeed, the plasma concentration and metabolism of both luteinizing hormone and follicle stimulating hormone are modified in animals and man by both acute and chronic ethanol administration.[85] The time courses of the changes are quite complex. Badr, Bartke, Dalterio and Bulger[86] found that depressions of plasma testosterone levels in mice were significant 30, 60 or 90 min after intragastric (introduced directly into the stomach) ethanol administration — a normal plasma titre was established 120 min after exposure. In contrast, although no changes in plasma luteinizing hormone were detected 3 h after ethanol administration in humans[87] such effects are evident 6 h after application.[70] Although in acute studies testosterone is maximally suppressed at the peak blood-alcohol level, luteinizing hormone levels only show a depression in the descending portion of the blood-alcohol curve. It has also been claimed that although doses above 1g/kg inhibit the pituitary-gonadal axis, lower doses may stimulate luteinizing hormone and testosterone titres.[69]

Ethanol may have to be metabolised in order to produce its inhibitory effect on plasma testosterone titre which appears to be at the level of the rate-limiting step of sex-steroid production from pregnenolone.[88] The alcohol dehydrogenase inhibitor, pyrazole, attenuates the effects of ethanol on steroidogenesis in the intact animal.[81] Ethanol appears to modify the conversion of androgens to oestrogens and may increase liver 5α reductase activity which is involved in the transformation of testosterone to its dihydrotestosterone metabolite.

It is also, conversely, well established that sex steroids have effects on the rate-limiting alcohol dehydrogenase in animals with testosterone inhibiting and oestradiol stimulating this enzyme system.[89] Rates of alcohol clearance from blood may also be influenced by reproductive processes such as lactation.[90]

The nature of the relationship between alcohol administration and plasma testosterone may be influenced by the population from which the sample is taken. Gordon, Southren, Vittek and Lieger[83] claimed that normal volunteers show 'a dampening of the episodic bursts of testosterone secretion followed by a fall in the plasma level of the steroid' over the first five days of alcohol application, and this was accompanied by increases in metabolic clearance rates. Greene and Hollander[91] note that 'hypogonadism (accompanied by impotence, testicular atrophy and sterility) and feminisation (with loss of male pattern of secondary sex hair, development of gynecomastia and vascular changes)' are commonly seen in male alcoholics. In contrast, the effects of alcoholism in gonadal function in females (on menstrual abnormalities, anovulation, signs of oestrogen deprivation in the uterus and the fallopian tubes and placental malfunction) are relatively limited. It is certainly true in individuals of both genders that alcohol could exert its actions at the level of the gonads, the pituitary or even the hypothalamus.

It is most pertinent to note speculation by Mendelson, Mello and Ellingboe[82] on the relationships between alcohol, testosterone secretion and human aggression. They claim that one needs clarification of (a) the precise temporal relationships between behaviour and the recorded hormonal changes seen during alcohol intoxication; and (b) evaluation of the effects of modifications of the hypothalamic/pituitary/gonadal axis during alcohol intoxication's effects on sexual and aggressive behaviours. One should note, however, that much of their speculation is based on a series of fallacies. 'Aggression' is *not* a unitary attribute, is *not* a uniquely masculine activity, and many forms of 'aggression' in animals and man are *not* particularly influenced by androgenic steroids.[79] This oversimplification seems to be due to a tendency to concentrate upon male organisms under a defined set of circumstances in aggression research.

Ethanol and Prostaglandins. Prostaglandins are hormone-like substances found in a variety of tissues including seminal fluid and the lungs. Prostaglandin E1 is said to possibly mediate some of the effects of ethanol, as alcohol may alter the production of this substance[92] which, in turn, has influences on platelet activity.[93]

Relating the Effects of Alcohol on Neurophysiology and Endocrinology to its Influence on Behaviour

Some of the problems of relating alcohol's effects on components of the neural and endocrine systems to changes in 'aggression' are emphasised in Figure 2.5.

The diagram attempts to show an interaction involving two participants viewed by an 'external' observer (NB this is not the only meaningful way of looking at 'aggression' in man). The first thing to note is that many of the behavioural components contributing to the social interaction are expressions of situational determinants. Another factor worth reiterating is that 'aggression' is only a part (often a minor part in terms of time allocated to it) of that interaction, and that the designation is at least partially determined by the history, status and preferences of the observer. Components of the neuroendocrine coordinating system (hormones and neurotransmitters, for example) which can to a certain extent modulate such interactions may express their effects through changed signalling between the participants (e.g. production of odours or sounds), changed perception of the situation/other individual, or by altered motivation (i.e. the individual's 'aggressiveness' or 'fearfulness'). As alcohol exerts very wide-ranging and complex effects upon aspects of neurophysiology and hormone production/degradation, it might be expected to alter any or all of these processes in the same or differing situations. One should also note that recorded social interactions are dynamic events (with arbitrary beginnings and ends), and the experiences gained from such encounters might be expected to alter physiology and/or subsequent behaviour. The time-course of ethanol's effects is also likely to be of particular importance.

The impression should be gained from the above that alcohol is not a 'magic bullet' that stimulates aggression — this is hardly remarkable as aggression is certainly *not* a condition like measles, mumps or syphilis. Disturbance of the system in one aspect is bound to have behavioural effects elsewhere. Changing components of the physiology must have repercussions throughout the entire organism. These points obviously cast considerable doubt

Figure 2.5: Complexities Inherent in Attempts to Relate CNS and Endocrine Activities to Aggression

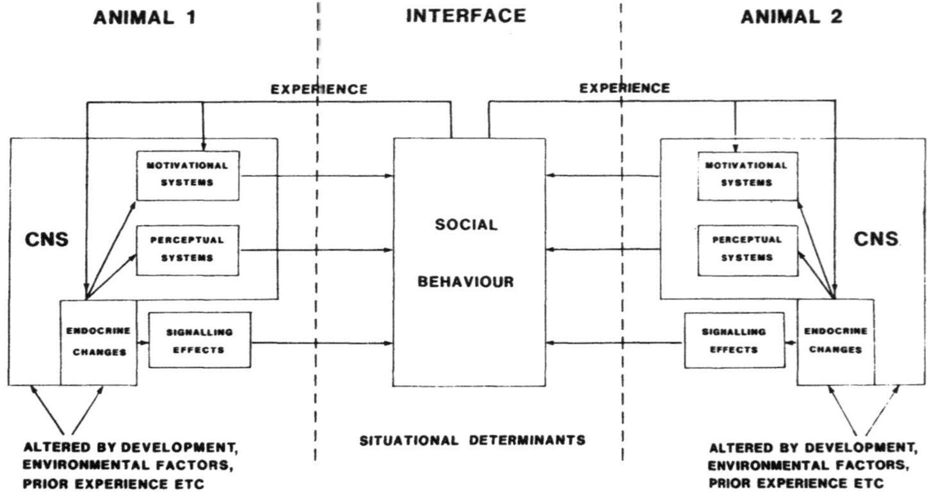

Note: This figure emphasises that the involvement of the neuroendocrine coordinating system in a social interaction can be extremely complex. The first thing to note is that the behaviour which is observed is social interaction, and 'aggression' is only a part of this (it is moreover a part which at least partially depends on the judgement of the external observer). The type of social behaviour is much influenced by situational determinants. The coordination systems of Animals 1 and 2 are represented in strongly diagrammatic forms, but at least three types of phenomena (involving neurons or hormones) can be identified. The coordination system may alter the 'aggression' component of the social encounter: (i) by changing motivation (most directly expressed as altered 'aggressiveness'); (ii) by modifying production of signals (odours, sounds or visual cues) passed between the interacting animals; or (iii) by altering the organism's perceptual systems so that they respond differently to particular signals. *All* necessarily input to behaviour. Furthermore, the situation is dynamic, which means that experiences gained in the social encounters feed-back to the organism's physiology, generating modifications of neural and endocrine function (leading to altered behaviour). Although the system illustrated is symmetrical, such symmetry is unlikely to persist as animals attain a dominance/subordination or a territory holder/intruder relationship. The point at issue is that all the types of input are possible and the system is highly integrated.

on the validity of the claim that 'booze' invariably results in aggression — it can, as is well known, result in joy, sexual arousal, despondency or sleep.

Conclusions

A somewhat reductionist approach has necessarily been taken in this chapter: the effects of alcohol have been described on single cells, discrete brain areas and individual endocrine systems. This is because most of our information and understanding are at this level. It should be remembered, however, that no cell, gland or brain nucleus in vertebrates acts independently. Similarly, aggression is only one (often limited) aspect of an animal's behavioural repertoire, and other activities will influence and be influenced by it. Aggression and other behavioural features are not neurochemically or even cerebrally organised as single entities within the brain (i.e. regions, groups of neurons or neurotransmitter systems).[94,95] Our understanding of alcohol-brain-aggression relationships seems likely to be most rapidly advanced by the use of ethological studies that quantify all behaviours and do not focus exclusively on aggression, and neurophysiological approaches that use a wide range of indices of brain function (from single-cell studies to electroencephalograms).

References

1. Gilman, A.G., Goodman, L.S. and Gilman, A. (eds) *The Pharmacological Basis of Therapeutics*, London: MacMillan, 1980.

2. Woodbury, J.W., D'Arrigo, J.S. and Eyring, H. 'Molecular mechanism of general anesthesia: Lipoprotein conformation change theory' in *Molecular Mechanisms of Anesthesia* (ed. Fink, B.R.); *Progress in Anesthesiology* vol. I, New York: Raven Press, 1975, pp. 253-75.

3. Erickson, C.K. 'Requirements for an ideal alcohol antagonist' in *Biological Effects of Alcohol* (ed. Begleiter, H.); *Advances in Experimental Medicine and Biology* vol. 126, 1980, 551-9.

4. Sun, A.Y. 'Biochemical and biophysical approaches in the study of ethanol-membrane interaction' in *Biochemistry and Pharmacology of Ethanol*, vol. 2 (eds Majchrowicz, E. and Noble, E.P.), New York: Plenum Press, 1979, pp. 81-99.

5. Pentreath, V.W. and Berry, M.S. 'Ethanol induces bursting amongst electrically coupled snail neurons', *Journal of Pharmacy and Pharmacology*, 1978, *30*, 321-3.

6. Eidelberg, E. 'Acute effects of ethanol and opiates on the nervous system'

Research Advances in Alcohol and Drug Problems, 1975, *2*, 147-76.
7. Wallgren, H. and Barry, H. *Actions of Ethanol, vol. 1, Biochemical, Physiological and Psychological Aspects*, Amsterdam: Elsevier, 1970.
8. Lake, N., Yarborough, G.G. and Phyllis, J.W. 'Effects of ethanol on cerebral cortical neurons: Interactions with some putative transmitters', *Journal of Pharmacy and Pharmacology*, 1973, *25*, 582-4.
9. Wayner, M.J., Gawronski, D., Roubie, C. and Greenberg, I. 'Effects of ethyl alcohol on lateral hypothalamic neurons' in *Recent Advances in Studies of Alcoholism* (eds Mello, N.K. and Mendelson, J.H.), US Government Printing Office: Washington, DC, 1971, pp. 219-73.
10. Roth, S.H. 'Differential effects of anesthetics on neuronal activity' in *Progress in Anesthesiology*, vol. 2 (ed. Fink, B.R.), New York: Raven Press, 1980, pp. 119-28.
11. Berry, M.S. and Pentreath, V.W. 'The neurophysiology of alcohol' in *Psychopharmacology of Alcohol* (ed. Sandler, M.), New York: Raven Press, 1980, pp. 43-72.
12. Faber, D.S. and Klee, M.R. 'Actions of ethanol on neuronal membrane properties and synaptic transmission' in *Alcohol and Opiates: Neurochemical and Behavioural Mechanisms* (ed. Blum, K.), New York: Academic Press, 1977, pp. 41-63.
13. Wise, C.D. and Stein, L. 'Facilitation of behaviour by augmented release of norepinephrine from the medial forebrain bundle' in *Amphetamine and Related Compounds* (eds Costa, E. and Garattini, S.), New York: Raven Press, 1970.
14. Meyer-Lohmann, J., Hagenah, R., Hellweb, C. and Berecke, R. 'The action of ethyl alcohol on the activity of individual Renshaw cells', *Naunyn Schmiedebergs Archives of Pharmacology*, 1972, *272*, 131-42.
15. Gage, P.W. 'The effect of methyl, ethyl and n-propyl alcohol on neuromuscular transmission in the rat', *Journal of Pharmacology and Experimental Therapeutics*, 1965, *150*, 236-43.
16. Inoue, F. and Frank, G.B. 'Effects of ethyl alcohol on excitability and neuromuscular transmission in frog skeletal muscle', *British Journal of Pharmacology and Chemotherapeutics*, 1967, *30*, 186-93.
17. Davidoff, R.A. 'Alcohol and presynaptic inhibition in an isolated spinal cord preparation', *Archives of Neurology*, 1973, *28*, 60-3.
18. Gage, P.W. and Hubbard, J.I. 'An investigation of the post-tetanic potentiation of end plate potentials at a mammalian neuromuscular junction', *Journal of Physiology (London)*, 1966, *184*, 353-75.
19. Woodson, P.B.J., Traynor, M.E., Schlapfer, W.T. and Barondes, S.H. 'Increased membrane fluidity implicated in acceleration of decay of post-tetanic potentiation by alcohols', *Nature*, 1976, *260*, 797-9.
20. Hess, W.R. *The Functional Organisation of the Diencephalon*, New York: Grune & Stratton, 1957.
21. Ursin, H. 'Neuroanatomical basis of aggression' in *Multidisciplinary Approaches to Aggression Research* (eds Brain, P.F. and Benton, D.), Amsterdam: Elsevier, 1981, pp. 269-93.
22. MacDonnell, M.F. and Ehmer, J. 'Some effects of ethanol on aggressive behaviour in cats', *Quarterly Journal of Studies on Alcohol*, 1969, *30*, 312-19.
23. MacDonnell, M.F. and Fessock, L. 'Some effects of ethanol, amphetamine, disulfiram and p-CPA on seizing of prey on feline predatory attack and on associated motor pathways', *Quarterly Journal of Studies on Alcohol*, 1972, *33*, 437-50.
24. Wasman, M. and Flynn, J.P. 'Directed attack elicited from the hypothalamus', *Archives of Neurology*, 1962, *6*, 220-7.
25. MacDonnell, M.F., Fessock, L. and Brown, S.H. 'Aggression and

associated neural events in cats: Effects of p-chlorophenylalanine compared with alcohol', *Quarterly Journal of Studies on Alcohol*, 1971, *32*, 748-63.

26. Johansson, G.G. 'Neural stimulation as a means of generating standardised threat under laboratory conditions' in *Multidisciplinary Approaches to Aggression Research* (eds Brain, P.F. and Benton, D.), Amsterdam: Elsevier, 1981, pp. 93-100.

27. Bandler, R. 'Neural control of aggressive behaviour', *Trends in Neuroscience*, 1982, *5*, 390-4.

28. Karli, P. 'Brain mechanisms underlying aggressive behaviour: a re-evaluation', *Trends in Pharmacology*, 1981, *2*, 285-6.

29. Delgado, J.M.R. 'Neuronal constellations in aggressive behaviour' in *Aggression and Violence: A Psychobiological and Clinical Approach* (eds L. Valzelli and L. Morgese), Edizioni St Vincent (Italy), 1981, pp. 82-98.

30. Blanchard, D.C., Blanchard, R.J., Takahashi, L.K. and Takahashi, T. 'Septal lesions and aggressive behavior', *Behavioral Biology*, 1977, *21*, 157-61.

31. Mendelson, J.H. 'Ethanol-1-C^{14} metabolism in alcoholics and non-alcoholics', *Science*, 1968, *159*, 319-20.

32. Leblanc, A.E., Kalant, H. and Gibbins, R.J. 'Acute tolerance to ethanol in the rat', *Psychopharmacologia*, 1975, *41*, 43-6.

33. Littleton, J.M. 'Biochemical aspects of alcohol tolerance and dependence' in *Pharmacological Treatments for Alcoholism* (eds Edwards, G. and Littleton, J.), London: Croom Helm, 1984, pp. 119-44.

34. Chin, J.H. and Goldstein, D.B. 'Drug tolerance in biomembranes: A spin label study of the effects of ethanol', *Science*, 1976, *196*, 684-5.

35. Ritzmann, R.F. and Tabakoff, B. 'Dissociation of alcohol tolerance and dependence', *Nature*, 1976, *263*, 418-20.

36. Shaw, G.K. 'Alcohol and the nervous system' in *Clinics in Endocrinology and Metabolism* vol. 7 (eds V. Marks and J. Wright), London: Saunders, 1978, pp. 385-405.

37. Walker, D.W., Barnes, D.E., Riley, J.N., Hunter, B.F. and Zornetzer, S.F. 'Neurotoxicity of chronic alcohol consumption: An animal model' in *Psychopharmacology of Alcohol* (ed. Sandler, M.), New York: Raven Press, 1980, 17-31.

38. Lishman, W.A., Ron, M. and Acker, W. 'Computed tomography of the brain and psychometric assessment of alcoholic patients — a British study' in *Psychopharmacology of Alcohol* (ed. Sandler, M.), New York: Raven Press, 1980, pp. 33-41.

39. Goldman, H., Sapirstein, L.A., Murphy, S. and Moore, J.C. 'Alcohol and regional blood flow in brains of rats', *Proceedings of the Society for Experimental Biology and Medicine*, 1973, *144*, 983-8.

40. Phillips, S.C. 'Does ethanol damage the blood brain barrier?', *Journal of Neurological Science*, 1981, *50*, 81-7.

41. Chin, J.H. 'Ethanol and the blood-brain barrier' in *Biochemistry and Pharmacology of Ethanol* vol. 2 (eds Majchrowicz, E. and Noble, E.P.), New York: Plenum Press, 1979, pp. 101-18.

42. Blunewicz, M.J., Dustman, R.E., Schenkenberg, T. and Beck, E.C. 'Neuropsychological correlates of chronic alcoholism and aging', *Journal of Nervous and Mental Disorders*, 1977, *165*, 348-55.

43. Ewing, J.A., Rouse, B.A. and Anderhold, R.M. 'Studies of the mechanism of Oriental hypersensitivity', *National Council on Alcoholism*, St Louis, 1978.

44. Melchior, C.L. 'Long-lasting effects of tetrahydroisoquinolines' in *Psychopharmacology of Alcohol* (ed. Sandler, M.), New York: Raven Press, 1980, pp. 149-53.

45. Sandler, M., Carter, S.B., Hunter, K.R. and Stern, G.M.

'Tetrahydroisoquinoline alkaloids: *In vivo* metabolites of L-DOPA in man', *Nature*, 1973, *241*, 439-43.

46. Cohen, G. and Collins, M.A. 'Alkaloids from catecholamines in adrenal tissue: Possible role in alcoholism', *Science*, 1970, *167*, 1749-51.

47. Pradhan, S.N. 'Aggression and central neurotransmitters', *International Review of Neurobiology*, 1975, *18*.

48. Pohorecky, L.A. and Jaffe, L.S. 'Noradrenergic involvement in the acute effects of ethanol', *Research Communications in Chemical and Pathological Pharmacology*, 1975, *12*, 433-47.

49. Carmichael, F.J. and Israel, Y. 'Effects of ethanol on neurotransmitter release by rat brain cortical slices', *Journal of Pharmacology and Experimental Therapeutics*, 1975, *193*, 824-34.

50. Littleton, J. 'Alcohol and neurotransmitters' in *Clinics in Endocrinology and Metabolism* vol. 7 (eds V. Marks and J. Wright), London: Saunders, 1978, pp. 369-84.

51. MacDonnell, M.F., Fessock, L. and Brown, S.H. 'Ethanol and the neural substrate for affective defense in the cat', *Quarterly Journal of Studies on Alcohol*, 1971, *32*, 406-19.

52. Sytinsky, T.A., Guzikov, B.M., Gomanko, M.V., Eremin, V.P. and Konovalova, N.N. 'The gamma-aminobutyric acid (GABA) system in brain during acute and chronic ethanol intoxication', *Journal of Neurochemistry*, 1975, *25*, 43-8.

53. Bayliss, W.M. and Starling, E.H. 'The mechanism of pancreatic secretion', *Journal of Physiology (London)*, 1902, *28*, 325-53.

54. Brain, P.F. 'Hormones and aggression in infra-human vertebrates' in *The Biology of Aggression* (eds Brain, P.F. and Benton, D.), Alphen aan den Rijn: Noordhoff/Sijthoff B.V., 1981, pp. 181-213.

55. Luttinger, D., Nemeroff, C.B., Mason, G.A., Frye, G.D., Breese, G.R. and Prange, A.J. 'Enhancement of ethanol-induced sedation and hypothermia by centrally administered neurotensin, β-endorphin and bombesin', *Neuropharmacology*, 1981, *20*, 305-9.

56. Little, H.J. and Wing, D.R. 'Alcohol' in *Psychopharmacology* vol. 1 (ed. D.G. Grahame-Smith), Amsterdam: Excerpta Medica, 1982, pp. 398-438.

57. Brain, P.F. 'Effects of the hormones of the pituitary-adrenocortical axis on behaviour' in *Chemical Influences on Behaviour* (eds Brown, K. and Cooper, S.J.), London: Academic Press, 1979, pp. 329-71.

58. McGivern, R.F., Harris, J.M., Yessaian, N., Kastin, A.J., Coy, D.H., Sandman, C.A. and Noble, E.P. 'Antagonism of ethanol induced sleep-time by d-MSH, MSH/ACTH 4-10 and naloxone', *Substance and Alcohol Actions/Misuse*, 1980, *1*, 335-42.

59. Ylikahri, R.H., Huttunen, M.O. and Harkonen, M. 'Hormonal changes during alcohol intoxication and withdrawal', *Pharmacology Biochemistry and Behavior*, 1980, *13* (Suppl. 1), 131-7.

60. Rudeen, P.K. and Symmes, S.K. 'Pineal gland and melatonin influence on chronic alcohol consumption by hamsters' *Pharmacology, Biochemistry and Behavior*, 1981, *14*, 143-8.

61. Van Thiel, D.H., Smith, W.F., Wight, C. and Abuid, J. 'Elevated basal and abnormal thyroid-releasing hormone-induced thyroid-stimulating hormone secretion in chronic alcoholic men with liver disease', *Alcohol: Clinical and Experimental Research*, 1979, *3*, 301-8.

62. Ylikahri, R.H., Huttunen, M.O., Harkonen, M., Leino, T., Helenius, T., Liewendahl, K. and Karonen, S.-L. 'Acute effects of alcohol on anterior pituitary secretion of the tropic hormones', *Journal of Clinical Endocrinology and Metabolism*, 1978, *46*, 715-20.

63. Peng, T.C. and Gitelman, H.J. 'Ethanol-induced hypocalcaemia, hypermagnesemia and inhibition of the serum calcium-raising effect of parathyroid hormone in rats', *Endocrinology*, 1974, *94*, 608-11.

64. Shah, J.H., Bowser, E.N., Hargis, G.K., Wongsurawat, N. Banerjee, P., Henderson, W.J. and Williams, G.A. 'Effects of ethanol on parathyroid hormone secretion in the rat', *Metabolism*, 1976, *27*, 257-60.

65. Janhonen, V.P. 'Effect of acute ethanol load on plasma immunoreactive insulin and glucagon', *Hormone and Metabolic Research*, 1978, *10*, 214-19.

66. McMonagle, J. and Felig, P. 'Effects of ethanol ingestion on glucose tolerance and insulin secretion in normal and diabetic subjects', *Metabolism*, 1975, *24*, 625-32.

67. Goas, J.A., Pelham, R.W. and Lippa, A.S. 'Endocrine factors contributing to the ethanol preferences of rodents', *Pharmacology, Biochemistry and Behavior*, 1979, *10*, 557-60.

68. Cobb, C.F., van Thiel, D.H., Gravaler, J.S. and Lester, R. 'Effects of ethanol and acetaldehyde on the rat adrenal', *Metabolism*, 1981, *30*, 537-43.

69. Kakihana, R. and Butte, J.C. 'Ethanol and endocrine function' in *Biochemistry and Pharmacology of Ethanol* vol. 2 (eds Majchrowicz, E. and Noble, E.P.), New York: Plenum Press, 1979, pp. 147-64.

70. Leppabioto, J., Rapeli, M., Varis, R. and Ranta, T. 'Secretion of anterior pituitary hormones in man: Effects of ethyl alcohol', *Acta Physiologica Scandinavica*, 1975, *95*, 400-6.

71. Hirvonen, J.I., Karlsson, L.K.J. and Ojala, K. 'Zum ein von Athanol auf die Zuna glomerulosa und Zuna fasciculata der Ratten-nebennierenrindebei gleichzeitiger Blastung mit Insulin und hypertonischer Kochsalzlosung', *Deutsche Zeitschrift für Gesamt die Gerichtliche Medizin* 1968, *62*, 232-8.

72. Lundy, J., Raaf, J.H., Deakins, S., Wanebo, H.J., Jacobs, D.A., Trung-dao, L., Jacobowitz, D., Spear, C. and Oettgen, H.F. 'The acute and chronic effects of alcohol on the immune system', *Surgery, Gynecology and Obstetrics*, 1975, *141*, 212-18.

73. Pohorecky, L.A. and Rizek, A.E. 'Biochemical and behavioral effects of acute ethanol in rats at different environmental temperatures', *Psychopharmacology*, 1981, *72*, 205-9.

74. Knych, E.T. and Prohaska, J.R. 'Effect of chronic intoxication and naloxone on the ethanol-induced increase in plasma corticosterone', *Life Sciences*, 1981, *28*, 1987-94.

75. Pohorecky, L.A., Rassi, E., Weiss, J.M. and Michalak, V. 'Biochemical evidence for an interaction of ethanol and stress: preliminary studies', *Alcoholism: Clinical and Experimental Research*, 1980, *4*, 423-6.

76. Green, V. 'Adrenal hormones and ethanol ingéstion in C57BL/Crgl and C3H/Crgl/2 mice', *Behavioral and Neural Biology*, 1981, *31*, 56-66.

77. Linkola, J., Fyhrquist, F., Nieminen, M.M., Weber, T.H. and Tontti, K. 'Renin-aldosterone axis in ethanol intoxication and hangover', *European Journal of Clinical Investigation*, 1976, *6*, 191-4.

78. Bourgeois, J.M. and Macabies, J. 'Depression by ethanol of the discharge of catecholamines induced by hypoglycemia in the dog', *Comptes Rendus des Sociétés de Biologie (Paris)*, 1974, *168*, 1029-33.

79. Brain, P.F., Haug, M. and vom Saal, F.S. 'Are female mice the docile sex?' in *The Aggressive Female* (eds Benton, D., Brain, P.F. and Haug, M.), Montreal: Eden Press, 1985.

80. Rubin, E., Lieber, C.S., Althan, K., Gary, G., Gordon, A. and Southren, A. 'Prolonged ethanol consumption increases testosterone metabolism in the liver', *Science*, 1976, *191*, 563-4.

81. Cicero, T.J., Newman, K.S. and Meyer, E.R. 'Ethanol-induced inhibitors

of testicular steroidogenesis in the male rat: mechanisms of actions', *Life Sciences*, 1981, *28*, 871-7.

82. Mendelson, J.H., Mello, N.K. and Ellingboe, J. 'Effects of alcohol on pituitary-gonadal hormones, sexual function and aggression in human males' in *Psychopharmacology: A Generation of Progress* (eds Lipton, M.A., Dimascio, A. and Killam, K.F.), New York: Raven Press, 1978, 1677-92.

83. Gordon, G.G., Southren, A.L., Vittek, J. and Lieger, C.S. 'The effect of alcohol ingestion on hepatic aromatase activity of plasma steroid hormones', *Metabolism*, 1979, *28*, 20-4.

84. Van Thiel, D.H., Gavaler, J.S., Cobb, C.F., Sherins, R.J. and Lester, R. 'Alcohol-induced testicular atrophy in the adult rat', *Endocrinology* 1979, *105*, 888-95.

85. Messiha, F.S. and Lox, C.D. 'The effect of acute and chronic administration of ethanol on circulating testosterone and luteinizing hormone secretion in the male rat', *Common Substance Abuse*, 1981, *2*, 117-26.

86. Badr, F.M., Bartke, A., Dalterio, S. and Bulger, W. 'Suppression of testosterone production by ethyl alcohol: Possible mode of action', *Steroids*, 1977, *30*, 647-55.

87. Toro, G., Kolodny, R.C., Jacobs, L.S., Masters, W.H. and Daughaday, W.H. 'Failure of alcohol to alter pituitary and target organ hormone levels', *Clinical Research*, 1973, *31*, p. 505.

88. Johnston, D.E., Chiao, Y.-B., Gavaler, J.S. and Van Thiel, D.H. 'Inhibition of testosterone synthesis by ethanol and acetaldehyde', *Biochemical Pharmacology*, 1981, *30*, 1827-32.

89. Rachamin, G., Macdonald, J.A., Wahid, S., Clapp, J.J., Khanna, J.M. and Israel, Y. 'Modulation of alcohol dehydrogenase and ethanol metabolism by sex hormones in the spontaneously hypertensive rat. Effect of chronic administration', *The Biochemical Journal*, 1980, *186*, 483-90.

90. Abel, E.L., Greizerstein, H.B. and Siemens, A.J. 'Influence of lactation on rate of disappearance of ethanol in the rat', *Neurobehavioral Toxicology*, 1979, *1*, 185-6.

91. Greene, L.W. and Hollander, C.S. 'Sex and alcohol: The effects of alcohol on the hypothalamic-pituitary-gonadal axis', *Alcoholism: Clinical and Experimental Research*, 1980, *4*, 1-5.

92. Manku, M.S., Oka, M. and Horrobin, D.F. 'Differential regulation of the formation of prostaglandins and related substances from arachidonic acid and from dihomogammalinolenic acid. I. Effects of ethanol', *Prostaglandins and Medicine*, 1979, *3*, p. 119.

93. Rotrosen, J., Mandio, D., Segarnick, D., Traficante, L.J. and Gershon, S. 'Ethanol and prostaglandin E_1: biochemical and behavioral interactions', *Life Sciences*, 1980, *26*, 1867-76.

94. Cools, A. 'Psychopharmacology and aggression: An appraisal of the current situation' in *The Biology of Aggression* (eds Brain, P.F. and Benton, D.), Alphen aan den Rijn: Noordhoff/Sijthoff, 1981, pp. 131-45.

95. Cools, A. 'Aspects and prospects of the concept of neurochemical and cerebral organisation of aggression: Introduction of new research strategies in "brain and behaviour" studies' in *The Biology of Aggression* (eds Brain P.F. and Benton, D.), Alphen aan den Rijn: Noordhoff/Sijthoff, 1981, pp. 405-25.

3 ALCOHOL AS A PSYCHOPHARMACOLOGICAL AGENT

Abdulla A.-B. Badawy

Introduction

Alcohol (ethanol) is a toxic agent capable of disturbing a wide variety of physiological functions, not only in the liver (where it is largely metabolised) but also elsewhere in the body. Ethanol causes these disturbances by one or more of the following four major mechanisms or actions (Table 3.1): (a) direct cytotoxicity (poisoning of cells); (b) pharmacological and neurochemical actions leading to the physiological and psychological changes characteristic of acute ethanol intoxication, alcohol dependence and the alcohol-withdrawal states; (c) disturbances secondary to alterations in endocrine function (whether these alterations are themselves caused by direct cytotoxic, or metabolic, mechanisms); (d) disturbances resulting from ethanol's own metabolism. The widespread occurrence in the body of these latter disturbances renders ethanol unique among drugs of dependence, and justifies a discussion in this chapter of ethanol metabolism and how it leads to these disturbances.

As in the case of most other pharmacological agents, the actions of alcohol (Table 3.2) depend on the dose administered or consumed, the species and/or strain of animal taking it, the route of its administration or intake and the time interval after intake and/or, in the human case, the state of alcoholism. In addition, the actions of alcohol are also influenced by differences in sex, genetic constitution and nutritional status, and by simultaneous exposure to other drugs. Many of the conflicting findings reported in the

Table 3.1: General Mechanisms of Actions of Alcohol

(a)	Direct cytotoxicity
(b)	Pharmacological and neurochemical actions
(c)	Disturbed endocrine function
(d)	Metabolic disturbances

literature concerning the biological actions of ethanol could be explained on the basis of these differences, emphasising the need for the strictest consideration of the above factors both in designing future experiments and interpreting their results. An important point one should stress at this stage is that the actions of alcohol vary depending on the state of its intake. For example, the effects on a particular biological phenomenon of an acute single dose of alcohol given to a naïve animal or to a human who is not a regular drinker may or may not be observable in a chronic alcohol-treated rat or a chronic alcoholic or during alcohol withdrawal. Chronic alcohol intake could thus influence the biological response to an acute single dose of the drug. In cases in which chronic alcohol consumption abolishes or lessens the extent of the acute effect, tolerance is said by some pharmacologists to have developed towards this particular acute effect. To establish that such tolerance has indeed developed, it is important that the original acute effect (observed in the naïve individual) is restored in the chronic alcoholic subject by intake of a larger dose of alcohol. Another example of the influence of the state of alcoholism on the actions of ethanol is that, although the chronic effects of the drug generally wear off either abruptly or gradually after withdrawal or cessation of intake, some of these effects may be replaced by new ones, or may even be altered in the opposite direction in the alcoholic organism.

The study of the relationship, if any, between the biological actions of alcohol and aggressive behaviour induced by its acute or chronic consumption or during subsequent withdrawal is also subject to the influences on these actions of the many factors and variables discussed above. The association is made even more difficult by the fact that very little is known about the biological or biochemical basis, particularly that related to central nervous system

Table 3.2: Factors Influencing the Actions of Alcohol

(a)	Dose consumed or administered
(b)	Species and/or strain of animal (or human race)
(c)	Route of intake or administration
(d)	Time interval, duration and state of intake or alcoholism
(e)	Sex differences
(f)	Genetic constitution
(g)	Nutritional status
(h)	Concomitant intake of other drugs

function, of aggressive behaviour or indeed behaviour in general. In view of the present state of knowledge in this area, it would therefore be clearly inappropriate (and perhaps meaningless) to ask the question which neurotransmitter or amine system in the brain is related to aggressive behaviour? Indeed, a similar question is also raised often when one tries to relate brain biochemistry to certain other disorders of the central nervous system, such as depressive illness or schizophrenia; and an appropriate answer, which also applies to aggression, would be that alterations in the brain functions of behaviour and mood probably represent changes in brain homeostasis involving many, if not all, neurotransmitter and amine systems and possibly also basic cellular (including membrane-related) mechanisms. However, despite these limitations, evidence has already emerged which suggests that behaviour can be related to changes in brain chemicals such as acetylcholine (AcCh), γ-aminobutyric acid (GABA), 5-hydroxytryptamine (5-HT or serotonin) and the catecholamines dopamine (DA) and noradrenaline (NA). The reader may wish to consult some recent publications for detailed accounts[1,2] of such evidence (which will be considered briefly later) and also of general reviews[3,4] of the relationship between alcohol and aggression.

It therefore appears from the above preamble that our knowledge of the relationship between the alcohol-induced aggressive behaviour and the biological actions of this drug is at a very preliminary stage. The present chapter can only therefore attempt to present to the reader an account of the actions of ethanol and its metabolism on some biological processes, particularly those thought to be related to mood and behaviour. No attempt will be made to discuss in any detail the influence of alcohol on neurophysiological and endocrine functions (see Chapter 2).

Ethanol Metabolism

Ethanol is metabolised mainly in the liver. It is thought that up to 20 per cent of a given dose of the drug may be metabolised extrahepatically (outside the liver). Ethanol metabolism has been the subject of much investigation and many reviews (for recent reviews and other publications, see refs 5, 6, 7 and 8), but, as stated in the introduction, the far-reaching metabolic consequences of ethanol oxidation justify a discussion here of this process and its consequences.

Ethanol Metabolism in vitro

There are three main enzyme systems capable of metabolising ethanol *in vitro* in liver preparations. These enzyme systems are alcohol dehydrogenase (ADH), catalase and the so-called microsomal ethanol-oxidising system (MEOS). These three enzyme systems resemble one another only in one respect; their ability to oxidise ethanol to acetaldehyde, according to the following three reactions:

$$CH_3CH_2OH + NAD^+ \xrightarrow{\text{ADH}} CH_3CHO + NADH + H^+$$

$$CH_3CH_2OH + H_2O_2 \xrightarrow{\text{Catalase}} CH_3CHO + 2H_2O$$

$$\underset{\text{ethanol}}{CH_3CH_2OH} + NADPH + H^+ + O_2 \xrightarrow{\text{Meos}} \underset{\text{acetaldehyde}}{CH_3CHO} + NADP^+ + 2H_2O$$

These three enzyme systems differ in many respects, including subcellular compartmentation and cofactor (coenzyme) requirements. Thus ADH is cytosolic (contained in the cytoplasm of the cell), MEOS, as its name implies, is microsomal and catalase has a wider distribution (being cytosolic, microsomal and peroxisomal). Also, whereas the catalase reaction does not require a cofactor, that of ADH utilises NAD^+ (oxidised nicotinamide-adenine dinucleotide) and MEOS uses NADPH (reduced nicotinamide-adenine dinucleotide phosphate).

The acetaldehyde produced by any of the above three reactions is then oxidised to acetate by the largely mitochondrial enzyme aldehyde dehydrogenase (AlDH), which, like ADH, requires NAD^+ as a cofactor, and catalyses the following reaction:

$$\underset{\text{Acetaldehyde}}{CH_3CHO} + NAD^+ + H_2O \xrightarrow{\text{AlDH}} \underset{\text{acetic acid}}{CH_3COOH} + NADH + H^+$$

The acetate produced as a result of ethanol oxidation by any one of the former three enzyme systems plus the AlDH reaction enters the common acetate pool to be further oxidised to carbon dioxide and water along the Krebs (tricarboxylic acid or citric acid) cycle, which is a biochemical process associated with the production of chemical energy. This is why alcohol intake provides energy, in the form of so-called 'empty calories', and this is the reason why severely chronic alcoholic subjects do not require as many calories from (and therefore consume less) food than non-alcoholics, with the result that malnutrition, vitamin deficiencies and related disorders become prevalent in such alcoholics.

A glance at the ADH and AlDH reactions described above will readily show that, in addition to the oxidation of ethanol to acetaldehyde and of the latter to acetate, NADH is produced by both reactions. As will be discussed later, this production of NADH, at the expense of NAD^+, is the most important biochemical event in alcohol metabolism in relation to intermediary and certain other metabolic processes in the body.

Ethanol Metabolism in vivo

As *in vitro*, the major enzyme systems likely to be involved in ethanol metabolism *in vivo* are ADH, catalase and MEOS. The abundance of catalase and the widespread occurrence of peroxidative reactions in the body have both led to the notion that catalase may play an active role in ethanol oxidation *in vivo*. Investigators have, however, failed to demonstrate such a role,[9,10] and this is because the catalase reaction is normally limited by the rate of generation of hydrogen peroxide.[11] This rate in rat liver *in vivo* is so small[12] that it can account for only 2 per cent of the rate of ethanol metabolism.[13] This does not, however, exclude the possibility[14] that, under certain pathological conditions (e.g. those involving increased purine breakdown), catalase may play a more active ethanol-oxidising role *in vivo*. The possibility that catalase could also play a more active role in ethanol oxidation *in vivo* under conditions of chronic alcohol consumption or chronic alcoholism is a controversial one (see ref. 5) and appears to be unsubstantiated by recent evidence.[15]

As regards MEOS, it now appears[16] that despite earlier controversy concerning its identity and function(s) (see refs 5 and 6 and references cited in both), it makes a more significant contribution (5-20 per cent, depending on experimental condition) than does catalase (2 per cent) to the overall rate of metabolism of ethanol *in vivo*. An active role for MEOS has recently received considerable support[17,18,19,20] from a variety of experimental approaches. MEOS may also be of importance in relation to alcohol tolerance, alcohol-drug interactions[16,17] and the area of toxicology in general.[17] This enzyme can be induced by chronic administration or consumption of ethanol and other drugs, and further work on these aspects may be of considerable interest.

As discussed previously,[5,6] there is universal agreement that ADH is quantitatively the most important enzyme of ethanol metabolism *in vivo*; this is further supported by more recent evidence.[7,19,21,22] As stated earlier, ethanol is metabolised mainly in the liver, but up to 20 per cent of the total body oxidation in man is extrahepatic.[23] In the rat, ADH activity is highest in the liver, with that of the second most active tissue (gastric mucosa) being only 3 per cent of that of the liver enzyme.[24] There is very little ADH activity in kidney cortex, testis and uterus, and almost none in lung, pancreas or spleen.[24] The brain contains some ADH,[25] but its activity is only 1/4000 of that of the liver enzyme and, consequently, this material is unlikely to be of any quantitative significance in relation to the overall rate of disposal of ethanol in the body.

Rate of Ethanol Metabolism in vivo

The rate of ethanol metabolism *in vivo* has been determined in man and experimental animals by a variety of methods,[5,6] the most widely used of which is that involving monitoring the rate of disappearance of ethanol from the blood. Although this disappearance rate can be shown to reflect ethanol metabolism, it should be remembered that clearance rate also depends on other factors, such as blood flow rates and the distribution of water in the body. The maximum rate of disappearance of ethanol from the blood of man is normally approximately 15mg/dl per hour. As will be discussed later, this is important to remember in relation to acute alcohol intoxication.

Factors Influencing Ethanol Metabolism

As discussed previously,[5,6] there are many factors that are known, or claimed, to influence ethanol metabolism *in vivo* and which could be classified generally into four major categories: (a) genetic differences; (b) chronic ethanol consumption; (c) NAD^+ availability; (d) other miscellaneous factors. It is now well recognised that genetic differences in the isoenzymes of ADH and AlDH are responsible for the differences known to exist between individuals and races in the rate of ethanol metabolism and in the sensitivity of persons to acute and chronic intake of the drug.[26,27,28] It has also been recognised for some 77 years[29] that chronic alcohol consumption accelerates ethanol metabolism. The mechanism of this effect has been the subject of much investigation,[5,6,17,19] and it is now generally believed that this could be explained by chronic ethanol consumption enhancing ADH activity to some extent, and (more significantly perhaps) by causing induction of synthesis of the microsomal ethanol-oxidising system MEOS. As stated earlier in this chapter, this MEOS induction could provide an explanation for alcohol tolerance.

The above miscellaneous group of factors (d) could be generally described as nutritional (starvation and under-nutrition, foodstuffs, vitamins and hormones), physical and physiological (exercise, hypothermia, shock, high temperature, cold exposure, high-altitude and high-oxygen tension) and pharmacological (psychoactive drugs). Apart from the influence on ethanol metabolism of certain foodstuffs such as fructose, which will be discussed below, and of nicotinamide and certain hormones and drugs, which all merit further investigation, studies on the possible efficacy of the remainder of the factors listed in this miscellaneous category have led to contradictory results.

There is overwhelming evidence[5,6,20,21,22,30] that availability or regeneration of liver NAD^+ appears to be the most important factor influencing ethanol metabolism by ADH. This is true whether regeneration involves the direct oxidation of free or ADH-bound NADH in the cytosol, or the indirect oxidation of cytosolic NADH in the mitochondria. NAD^+ availability in the hepatic cytosol becomes an important factor in ethanol metabolism (particularly when the amount of ethanol reaching the liver exceeds the rate of its oxidation therein), because achievement of the latter by the catalytic action of cytosolic ADH leads to a deficiency in free cytosolic $[NAD^+]$ as a result of its reduction to NADH. The resultant decrease in cytosolic $[NAD^+]$ becomes an acute intracellular problem that cannot be corrected rapidly by the liver. This is largely because the mitochondrial membranes are impermeable to NAD^+ and NADH, such that cytosolic NADH cannot cross into the mitochondria (where it can easily be oxidised), and mitochondrial NAD^+ (produced in abundance as part of the electron-transport function of these organelles) is not capable of easy exit into the cytosol. Under these conditions the liver can achieve a limited degree of success in regenerating cytosolic NAD^+ by a number of mechanisms. Thus cytosolic NADH can be oxidised to NAD^+ by reacting with substrates of certain cytosolic dehydrogenases, such as pyruvate and dihydroxyacetone phosphate. Alternatively, NADH bound to ADH can be oxidised directly in the cytosol by substances such as glyceraldehyde, which is a metabolite of the sugar fructose. The usefulness of this sugar in accelerating ethanol metabolism during acute alcohol intoxication is therefore based on this mechanism and also on another involving direct oxidation of free cytosolic NADH through the provision of another metabolite, pyruvate. The third mechanism by which the liver can regenerate cytosolic NAD^+ is that of indirect oxidation of cytosolic NADH in the mitochondria by the action of the so-called 'substrate shuttle' systems[6] (see Figure 3.1). Briefly, because cytosolic NADH cannot enter the mitochondria, its oxidation in these organelles is achieved through the movement across the mitochondrial membranes of substrates and products of certain NAD^+-linked dehydrogenases which must be present in both cytosol and mitochondria. For example, taking the most important shuttle system, the malate-aspartate shuttle, the following sequence of events can be drawn: (a) the excess NADH in the cytosol (resulting from ethanol metabolism) favours the conversion of oxaloacetate to malate by the cytosolic malate dehydrogenase reaction; (b) malate enters the mitochondria and becomes oxidised to oxaloacetate by the action of mitochondrial malate dehydrogenase in the presence of NAD^+; (c) oxaloacetate exits from the mitochondria into the cytosol (indirectly, because of a permeability problem) as aspartate (after transamination), which is then back-transaminated to oxaloacetate in the cytosol; (d) oxaloacetate in the cytosol is finally reduced to malate during the malate dehydrogenase reaction, using the excess NADH, thus regenerating NAD^+ in the cytosol.

Acute ethanol intoxication occurs when blood-ethanol concentration exceeds 80mg/dl. Under these conditions alcohol depresses the central nervous system, thus impairing many functions, because it accumulates in the blood at a rate faster than that of its removal from the circulation (15mg/dl/hr), which is determined largely by metabolism in the liver. A person whose blood-ethanol concentration is 80mg/dl will therefore require approximately 5 hours before achieving total elimination of ethanol from the circulation. Since the above three mechanisms by which NAD^+

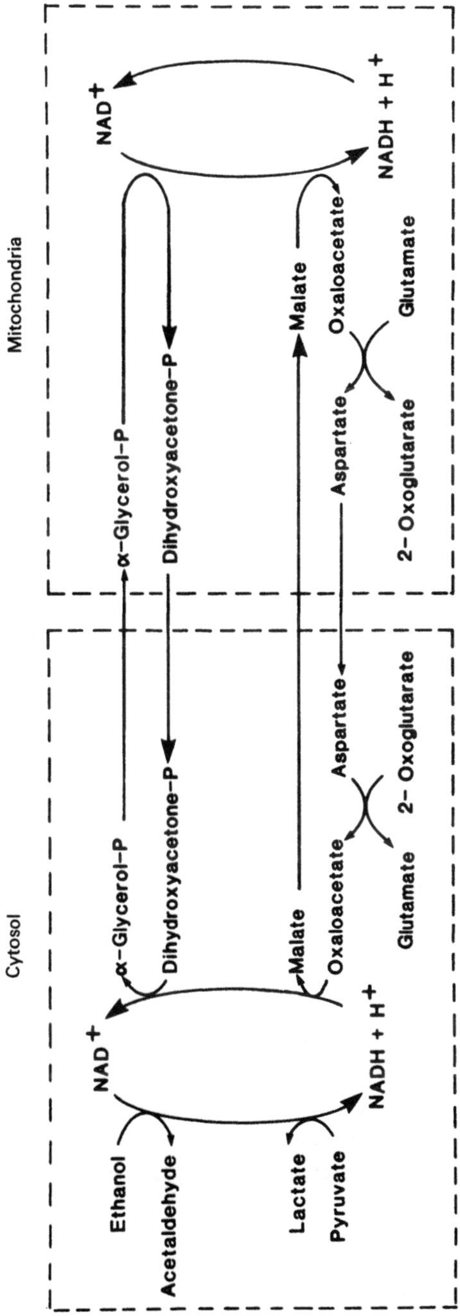

Figure 3.1: The Role of the Substrate Shuttles in Hepatic Ethanol Metabolism

can be regenerated into the cytosol are not fast enough to achieve rapid elimination of ethanol from the blood, the successful treatment of acute alcohol intoxication must rely on external measures, aimed at either counteracting the central nervous system depressing actions of ethanol (pharmacodynamic antagonism) and/or accelerating ethanol metabolism or elimination (pharmacokinetic antagonism). An account of compounds antagonising acute ethanol intoxication by these mechanisms has been published by Alkana and Noble,[31] who coined the term 'amethystic agents' to describe them. One agent that promises to be an accelerator of ethanol metabolism as well as being a pharmacodynamic antagonist of acute alcohol intoxication is the opiate receptor antagonist naloxone.[32]

Implications of Ethanol Metabolism for Intermediary and other Metabolic Processes

As stated earlier in this section, the increased formation of NADH during ethanol oxidation by ADH is the most important result of alcohol metabolism, because this increase, which leads to a decrease in the ratio of $[NAD^+]/[NADH]$, has far-reaching implications for intermediary and other metabolic processes.[33] This is because most of these processes are NAD^+-dependent, and any disturbances in the free $[NAD^+]/[NADH]$ ratio can therefore disturb the equilibrium known to exist between this redox (oxidation-reduction) ratio and that of substrates of NAD^+-linked dehydrogenases. For example, in the hepatic cytosol, where the primary disturbance of the $[NAD^+/[NADH]$ ratio occurs, there is an equilibrium between this redox pair and the substrates of lactate dehydrogenase, malate dehydrogenase and α-glycerophosphate dehydrogenase. Thus, when [NADH] is increased in the cytosol as a result of ethanol metabolism by alcohol dehydrogenase, the equilibria of the above three enzymes are disturbed such that all three reactions proceed in the direction of reduction, as follows:

$$\text{NADH} + \text{H}^+ + \text{pyruvate} \longrightarrow \text{NAD}^+ + \text{lactate}$$
$$\text{NADH} + \text{H}^+ + \text{oxaloacetate} \longrightarrow \text{NAD}^+ + \text{malate}$$
$$\text{NADH} + \text{H}^+ + \text{dihydroxyacetone phosphate} \longrightarrow \text{NAD}^+ + \alpha\text{-glycerophosphate}$$

Many other disturbances occur as a result of alcohol intake and this leads to widespread disruption of metabolic processes in the body, with, in many cases, serious consequences. Although these disturbances are too numerous to list, it is, nevertheless, useful to briefly discuss some that may be relevant to the area of aggressive behaviour, namely: (a) glucose metabolism; (b) biogenic amine metabolism; (c) endocrine metabolism.

It is well known that alcohol intake induces hypoglycaemia (i.e. a low blood-sugar condition) mainly as a result of inhibition of gluconeogenesis (formation of glucose from non-carbohydrate sources) (for reviews, see refs 33 and 34). Hypoglycaemia impairs many nervous and other biological functions, causing irritability and perhaps leading to the development of aggressive behaviour. The increase in [NADH] caused by alcohol intake could also disturb the metabolism of biogenic amines, which are important regulators of mood and behaviour. For example, it is known[35,36] that the ethanol-induced increase in [NADH] and possibly also the associated production of acetaldehyde lead to a diversion of biogenic amine metabolism from the major oxidative pathway (that leading to production of biogenic acids) to the minor reductive pathway resulting in the formation of biogenic alcohols. In the case of 5-hydroxytryptamine (5-HT), this diversion facilitates the formation of large amounts of the biogenic alcohol 5-hydroxytryptophol, which induces sleep and exerts effects on behaviour in experimental animals. In addition, ethanol consumption leads to the formation in the brain and elsewhere in the body of complex compounds through interaction between biogenic amines and either acetaldehyde (produced from ethanol oxidation by alcohol dehydrogenase) or biogenic aldehydes, whose levels are also increased by the action of alcohol. These complex compounds (tetrahydro-β-carbolines and tetrahydroisoquinolines, formed respectively from 5-HT and the catecholamines) have been shown to be addictive and also to influence behaviour. It is not clear at present, however, if all these compounds (complex or otherwise) have an influence on behaviour leading to aggression, but it would be surprising if they did not, in view of their actions on mood and behaviour in general; further work in this area may therefore be fruitful. Alcohol also influences biogenic amine metabolism in other ways (which will be discussed in detail later on) which may have a more direct relationship with aggressive behaviour. Endocrine function can be disturbed by ethanol (for reviews, see refs 37, 38 and 39) and this too may be important in relation to aggressive behaviour, in view of the role(s) of hormones in the control of mood, emotion and other related biological phenomena and processes. As stated in the introduction, the effects of ethanol on endocrine function in relation to aggression will be considered in detail in Chapter 2, but it is sufficient to state here that, as well as by exerting a direct cytotoxic action and by influencing hormone release, ethanol alters endocrine function also by a metabolic mechanism(s) related to the ability of the disturbed $[NAD^+]/[NADH]$ ratio to influence the directions of reactions involved in hormone metabolism, such as those involved in steroidogenesis (Δ^4, Δ^5-isomerase, 3β-hydroxysteroid reductase and 17β-reductase) (see refs 37 and 39 and references cited in both).

Relationship Between Aggressive Behaviour and Brain Chemicals

As stated earlier, there are many limitations to our understanding of the neurochemical basis of aggressive behaviour or indeed any behaviour. These limitations are not only procedural, but also exist because conclusions derived from studies attempting to correlate aggressive behaviour with changes in brain chemicals could be influenced by a variety of factors,[40] notably the type of behaviour being investigated, the region of brain being examined, the specificity of action(s) of drugs used to modify neurochemical processes, drug-treatment schedules, genetic differences and stress and other environmental factors. However, despite these limitations, evidence suggesting that behaviour can be correlated with changes in brain chemicals such as acetylcholine (AcCh), γ-aminobutyric acid (GABA), 5-hydroxytryptamine (5-HT or serotonin) and the catecholamines dopamine (DA) and noradrenaline (NA) does exist. Other substances, such as trace amines and certain metabolites, may also be involved.[1] Much of this evidence has been derived from animal studies, and care must therefore be exercised in extrapolating to the human situation. This is not, however, to say that further animal studies will not be helpful in conjunction with human investigations of the biological basis of behaviour.

The above evidence has recently been discussed in detail elsewhere,[1,2] as has the relationship[3,4] between alcohol intake and aggressive behaviour. It may, however, be useful to summarise the above evidence before describing in detail the effects of ethanol on the above brain chemicals. Despite many conflicting findings, it can generally be concluded that aggressive behaviour is associated with decreases in concentrations, turnover rates or neuronal activities of 5-HT and GABA and with increases in those of AcCh. In the case of the catecholamines, aggression appears to depend on the balance between DA and NA, although it generally may be associated with a decrease in NA and an increase in DA. Here again, caution must be exercised in attributing any specific aggressive behaviour to any particular chemical, because of the accumulated evidence suggesting the existence of mutual interaction and control mechanisms influencing metabolism, release and functions of various brain amines and neurotransmitters. It is accordingly more profitable for the investigator to consider these interaction and control processes in interpreting any selective changes in a specific substance in relation to behaviour.

Ethanol and Brain γ-aminobutyric acid (GABA)

The actions of ethanol on brain GABA metabolism and functions, including the binding characteristics of the benzodiazepine-GABA receptor, have recently been reviewed.[41,42] Very little work has been done in this area and reported studies have led to contradictory conclusions. This is largely because of the different experimental conditions imposed and the limited observations made, particularly as regards the dose of, and duration of treatment with, ethanol. In addition, as pointed out by Hunt and Majchrowicz,[41] very few attempts have been made in studies on the effects of ethanol on GABA to distinguish between GABA as a metabolic intermediate and GABA as an inhibitory neurotransmitter. It is, nevertheless, possible to conclude that decreases in GABA concentration previously associated with aggressive behaviour accompany the increase in locomotor activity seen after acute administration of a small dose of ethanol, and also the seizures observed during the alcohol-withdrawal syndrome. Of additional interest are the findings[42] that numbers of low-affinity GABA receptor sites are decreased during alcohol withdrawal, and that this decreased affinity can be correlated with audiogenic-seizure activity. Very recently, Simler, Kempf, Puglisi-Allegra, Ciesielski and Mandel[43] reported that GABA concentrations in olfactory bulbs and striata of an inbred aggressive strain of mice are lower than in corresponding structures of brains of a non-aggressive strain. Apart from these studies, very little has been done to determine how ethanol influences GABA levels and metabolism and (more importantly perhaps) the effects (if any) of ethanol on GABA functions as an inhibitory neurotransmitter. Detailed biochemical investigations of these questions in conjunction with sophisticated behavioural analysis may prove very fruitful in this area.

Ethanol and Brain Acetylcholine (AcCh)

The effects of ethanol on the cholinergic system have been reviewed by Massarelli,[44] who emphasised the meagre and often contradictory literature on this subject. He claimed that, because of our poor knowledge of the rate-limiting step of acetylcholine turnover, the effects of ethanol reported must be viewed with caution as well as interest. These contradictory findings may be explained as resulting not only from the evident pharmacological and procedural differences (i.e. dose of ethanol and route and duration of its administration, etc.) and other methodological differences, but also the complex and integrated aspects of the control of metabolism and the functions of the cholinergic system. Despite these limitations it is possible to conclude that ethanol exerts a biphasic effect on the concentration of AcCh in the brain stem and the striatum, producing an increase acutely and a decrease after chronic treatment. Cholinergic transmission is also influenced by ethanol, with neuromuscular junctions being affected differently from nervous tissue. Thus, AcCh release is increased in motor end plates, but decreased in brain slices and the perfused brain. By contrast, the effects of ethanol on the enzymes of choline metabolism (e.g. choline acetyltransferase and acetylcholine esterase) are contraversial. This scanty information and the absence of any data on the possible relationship between the ethanol-induced aggressive behaviour and the drug effects on the cholinergic system render any conclusions concerning this relationship premature, but emphasise the need for further investigations.

Ethanol and Brain Catecholamines

Catecholamines have been much more extensively studied in relation to ethanol and behaviour than GABA and AcCh. The effects of ethanol on the metabolism and functions of catecholamines have recently been reviewed by Hunt and Majchrowicz.[41] They pointed out that the conflicting and controversial findings previously reported on this topic could be explained largely on the basis of methodological differences, the most important of which appear to be the dose of ethanol given, the route and duration of its administration and concomitant treatment with other drugs. Before detailing the effects of ethanol on catecholamine metabolism and functions, it may be useful to briefly discuss some aspects of metabolism of these amines, as this may have relevance to the mechanism(s) of action of ethanol.

Brain Catecholamine Synthesis and its Control

Catecholamines are synthesised from the aromatic amino acid *L*-tyrosine. This precursor amino acid is first hydroxylated to *L*-dopa (3,4-dihydroxyphenylalanine) by the action of the first and rate-limiting enzyme of the catecholamine-biosynthetic pathway, tyrosine hydroxylase. This *L*-dopa produced is then decarboxylated to form dopamine (3,4-dihydroxyphenethylamine) by the aromatic *L*-amino acid decarboxylase. Dopamine (DA) is then hydroxylated by dopamine-β-hydroxylase to form noradrenaline (NA). In addition to the rate-limiting control by tyrosine hydroxylase, brain catecholamine synthesis also appears controlled by the availability of the amino acid precursor tyrosine[45,46,47] because the above enzyme exists in neural material unsaturated with its tyrosine substrate. Brain catecholamine synthesis could therefore be influenced significantly by even minor[47] fluctuations in brain tyrosine concentration, and it follows that peripheral (as well as central) factors influencing tyrosine availability to, or within, the brain may exert an important effect on cerebral catecholamine synthesis. As will be seen later, the most important of these factors are the activity of liver tyrosine aminotransferase (quantitatively the most important enzyme of tyrosine catabolism in the body), and the influence of competing amino acids on cerebral uptake of circulating tyrosine.

Acute Effects of Ethanol

These effects have been reviewed up to 1979 by Hunt and Majchrowicz.[41] The acute effects of this drug on concentrations, turnover rates, uptake and release of catecholamines and also on behaviour in the presence of catecholamine-modifying agents are all variable and depend on the dose of, and time interval after, ethanol administration, as well as many other factors. Thus, brain catecholamine levels are elevated at 1 hour, but decreased at 2-6 hours, after ethanol administration. Turnover of DA and NA are also altered in parallel; with an early increase followed by an inhibition. Release of both catecholamines from slices of caudate nuclei was also influenced in a similar biphasic fashion: an initial increase (when blood-ethanol concentration was up to 300mg/dl) followed by an inhibition at higher blood-ethanol concentrations. A recent study[48] attempting to examine in detail the acute effects of ethanol on rat brain catecholamine synthesis and metabolism as a function of the dose of the drug and the time interval after its administration found (Figure 3.2) that a 4g/kg body wt dose of ethanol exerted the following effects: (a) an enhancement of catecholamine (DA and NA) synthesis at 1 hour associated with an increased brain tyrosine concentration and an enhancement of tyrosine hydroxylase activity (as assayed *in vitro*) and of the rate of tyrosine hydroxylation by the brain *in vivo*; (b) an inhibition of brain catecholamine synthesis at 2-4 hours associated with a decrease in brain tyrosine concentration; (c) a return of brain catecholamine synthesis to normal at 6 hours preceded 1 hour earlier by a decrease in serum competing (neutral) amino acids; (d) an enhancement of cerebral catecholamine synthesis at 8 hours associated with increased uptake of circulating tyrosine; (e) an inhibition of cerebral catecholamine synthesis at 12 hours associated with a decreased brain tyrosine concentration; (f) a final return of brain catecholamine synthesis to normal 16 hours after ethanol administration. All these alterations in brain catecholamine synthesis were mediated by corresponding changes in brain tyrosine concentration, providing considerable evidence to emphasise the important role of brain tyrosine in catecholamine synthesis. Additional studies[48,49,50,51] confirmed that the above multiple effects of acute ethanol administration on rat brain catecholamine synthesis and the corresponding alterations in brain tyrosine concentration were caused by this drug either influencing liver tyrosine aminotransferase activity and brain tyrosine transamination or affecting the level of serum amino acids competing with tyrosine for the same cerebral uptake mechanism. It was of particular interest that brain catecholamine synthesis[48] and the rate of transamination of tyrosine in the liver[50] were significantly influenced by a dose of ethanol as low as 0.2g/kg body wt, which is equivalent to one-half to one pint of commercial beer being consumed by a 70kg human.

Figure 3.2: Effects of Acute Ethanol Administration on Tyrosine Metabolism and Disposition in the Rat

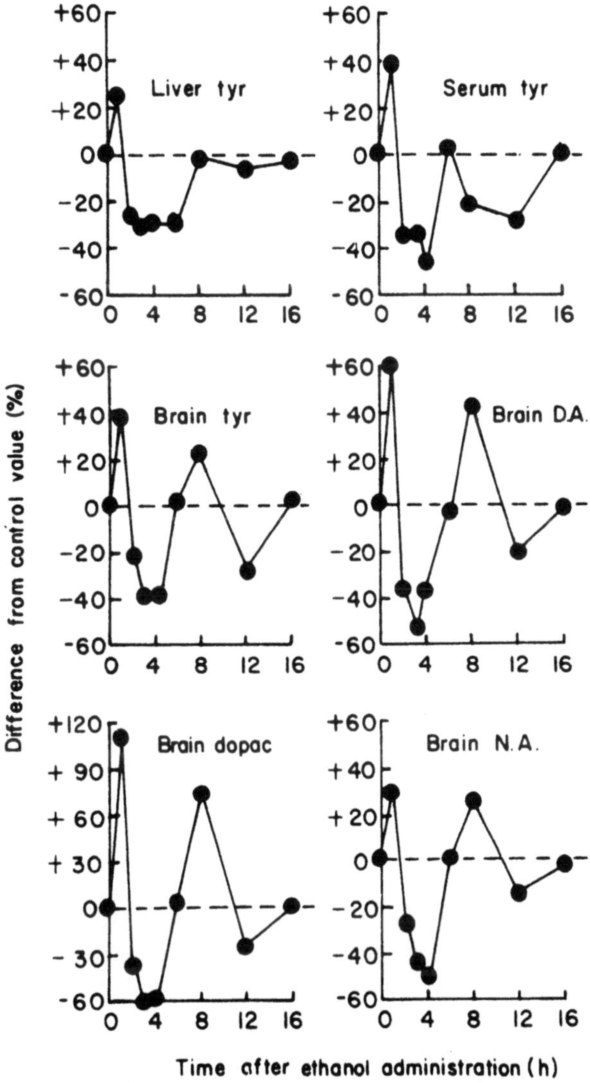

Note: Ethanol (4g/kg body wt) was administered intraperitoneally at zero-time. Control rats received an equal volume (20ml/kg) of saline. Abbreviations used: tyr (tyrosine); DA (dopamine: 3,4-dihyroxyphenethylamine); dopac (3,4-dihydroxyphenylacetic acid); NA (noradrenaline). This figure is reproduced here from ref. 48 by permission.

Chronic and Withdrawal Effects of Ethanol

In contrast to the acute effects, chronic ethanol administration or consumption or subsequent withdrawal have been less extensively studied and have generated more controversial findings (for a review, see ref. 41). Thus, concentrations of NA and DA in whole brain or certain brain areas have been reported to be unaltered, increased or decreased by chronic ethanol treatment, depending on the duration of intake. NA and DA turnover is known to be increased during chronic intake, whereas that of DA has been shown to be decreased during the alcohol-withdrawal syndrome. Release of DA from slices of caudate nuclei is enhanced after four days of ethanol intake, but is inhibited during withdrawal. In contrast to most of these metabolic findings, behavioural observations during chronic ethanol intake and subsequent withdrawal have been more consistent, with the withdrawal-induced convulsions and the associated increase in locomotor stimulation being respectively potentiated and inhibited by NA-modifying agents, whereas the convulsions are inhibited by DA and its precursor *L*-dopa. Clearly much more work is required, not only to examine precisely the nature and mechanism(s) of action(s) of chronic ethanol consumption and subsequent withdrawal on the metabolism and functions of brain catecholamines, but also to study the relationship(s) between these effects and changes in behaviour (especially aggression).

Ethanol and Brain 5-hydroxytryptamine (5-HT)

Because it has been implicated in the regulation of mood and behaviour and in the actions of drugs of dependence and other neurally active drugs, 5-HT has been of considerable interest to investigators of the actions of ethanol, and features prominently in current theories of alcoholism and also other forms of drug dependence. Indeed, the effects of acute and chronic ethanol administration and subsequent withdrawal on brain 5-HT metabolism have been extensively studied and recently reviewed.[41,52,53,54] As in the case of the catecholamines, studies of the effects of acute and chronic administration and subsequent withdrawal of ethanol on brain 5-HT metabolism and functions have led to conflicting findings. These appear largely due to differences in doses of ethanol, routes and durations of administration, species and/or strains of animals used and methods of assessment of certain aspects of 5-HT metabolism. Before describing in detail the actions of ethanol on brain 5-HT, it may be useful to briefly discuss the regulation of synthesis of this indoleamine and the role of tryptophan in this process, as this is important in relation to the above actions of ethanol.

Brain 5-HT Synthesis and its Control

Brain 5-HT is synthesised from the aromatic amino acid *L*-tryptophan. As in the case of catecholamine synthesis, the rate-limiting step of the 5-HT-biosynthetic pathway is the first step involving the hydroxylation of the amino acid by tryptophan hydroxylase. The product, 5-hydroxytryptophan, is then decarboxylated to form 5-HT. Because brain tryptophan hydroxylase exists normally unsaturated with its amino acid substrate, the synthesis of 5-HT is strongly influenced by changes in brain tryptophan concentration. It also follows that brain 5-HT synthesis can be influenced by peripheral factors known to affect tryptophan availability to the brain. These are: (a) the extent of binding of tryptophan to serum or plasma proteins;[55] (b) competition from neutral amino acids in plasma;[56] (c) the activity of the major tryptophan-degrading enzyme, liver tryptophan pyrrolase.[52,53,54,57,58]

Acute Effects of Ethanol

As stated previously,[41] acute studies of the effects of ethanol on brain 5-HT concentration, synthesis or turnover have led to contradictory findings. When methodological problems were considered in a detailed study,[52,59] it was found that the acute effects of ethanol on brain 5-HT synthesis depend mainly on the species and strain of animal, dose of ethanol and time interval after its administration. Thus (as shown in Figure 3.3), acute administration to male Wistar rats of a 4g/kg body wt dose of ethanol exerts a biphasic effect on tryptophan and 5-HT metabolism, with brain 5-HT synthesis (as assessed from changes in concentrations of 5-HT and its major metabolite 5-HIAA (5-hydroxyindol-3-yl acetic acid)) being initially enhanced but later inhibited. This biphasic effect on cerebral 5-HT synthesis is closely associated with corresponding changes in brain tryptophan concentration induced by parallel alterations in the availability of circulating free (i.e. non-protein-bound) tryptophan. The mechanisms by which acute ethanol administration exerts this biphasic effect on neural tryptophan availability were found[52,59] to consist of an initial displacement of serum protein-bound tryptophan by non-esterified fatty acids secondarily to enhancement of lipolysis (fat breakdown) by peripheral release of catecholamines, followed by a later decrease in tryptophan availability caused by increased hepatic degradation of the amino acid following from an enhancement of liver tryptophan pyrrolase activity, which is itself produced by the initial increase in availability (to the liver) of circulating free tryptophan.

5-HT uptake or release (by brain slices or synaptosomes) appears uninfluenced by ethanol *in vitro* or in ethanol-dependent rats (see ref. 41 and references cited therein).

Chronic and Withdrawal Effects of Ethanol

The effects of chronic ethanol consumption and subsequent withdrawal on brain 5-HT metabolism have been recently reviewed.[41,53,54] The contradictory literature in this area can be explained on the basis of the usual methodological differences and the use by most investigators of isocaloric doses of sucrose or glucose as control treatments (these have been shown[60] to mask the chronic effects of ethanol on 5-HT synthesis). When these points were considered, it was found[53,61,62,63] that chronic ethanol administration enhances, whereas subsequent withdrawal inhibits, rat brain 5-HT synthesis. The results summarised in Figure 3.4 show that chronic ethanol consumption increases the concentrations of brain 5-HT and 5-HIAA, whereas withdrawal of the drug causes the opposite changes. These opposite effects of chronic administration and subsequent withdrawal of ethanol on cerebral 5-HT synthesis appear to be caused by corresponding changes in brain tryptophan concentration elicited by corresponding alterations in the availability of circulating tryptophan to the brain. These latter alterations (see Figure 3.4) involve proportionate increases during chronic ethanol consumption and relative decreases during subsequent withdrawal in both free serum and total serum tryptophan concentrations. These proportionate changes, which are unassociated with any disturbance in tryptophan binding to serum proteins, usually indicate corresponding alterations in hepatic tryptophan degradation by tryptophan pyrrolase. Changes in hepatic tryptophan degradation are suggested to be the cause of the above opposite effects of chronic ethanol con-

Figure 3.3: Effects of Acute Ethanol Administration on Tryptophan Metabolism and Disposition in the Rat

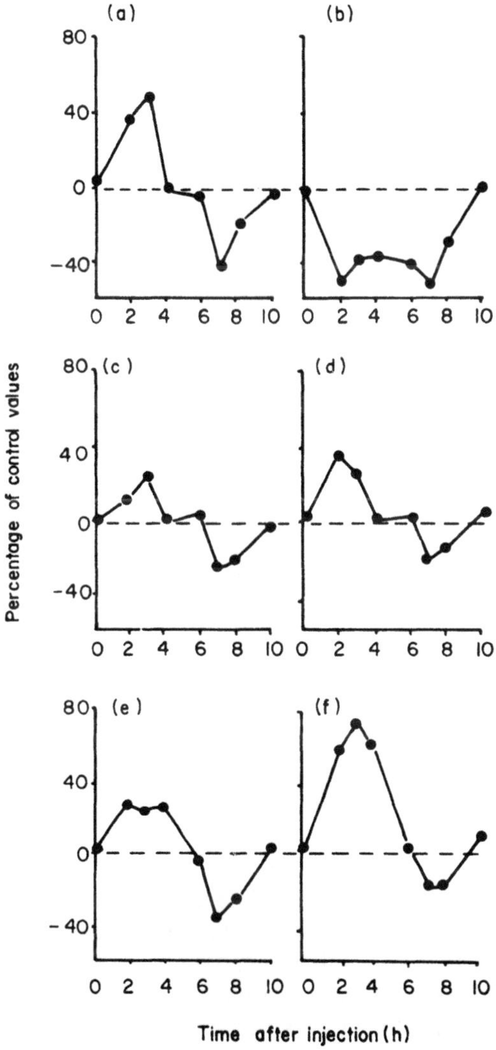

Note: Ethanol (4g/kg body wt) was administered intraperitoneally at zero-time. Control rats received an equal volume (20ml/kg) of saline. Symbols are: (a) free serum tryptophan; (b) total serum tryptophan; (c) liver tryptophan; (d) brain tryptophan; (e) brain 5-HT; (f) brain 5-HIAA. This figure is reproduced here from ref. 59 by permission.

sumption and subsequent withdrawal on circulating tryptophan availability by the observed (Figure 3.4) increase and decrease respectively in liver tryptophan concentration. It has been known for some time[64,65] that chronic ethanol administration inhibits, whereas subsequent withdrawal enhances, rat liver tryptophan pyrrolase activity, and that the inhibition elicited by chronic consumption has been shown to be caused by an increase in liver [NAD(P)H], whereas the enhancement observed during subsequent withdrawal is produced by a hormonal-type induction mechanism. In Figure 3.5, whereas liver total and apo-(tryptophan pyrrolase) activities are inhibited by chronic ethanol consumption, subsequent withdrawal induces a proportionate increase in all forms of the enzyme (i.e. a hormonal-type induction) with the maximal effects occurring eight days after withdrawal. Figure 3.5 also shows that this induction of liver tryptophan pyrrolase during alcohol withdrawal correlates with an increase in concentration of serum corticosterone, which is the major glucocorticoid (and pyrrolase inducer) in the rat. This increased release of corticosterone appears a feature of not only alcohol withdrawal, but also withdrawal of other drugs of dependence[57] and represents an important mechanism by which such compounds influence brain biochemistry and possibly also behaviour.

Summary, Conclusions and Comments

It is clear that acute and chronic ethanol administration or intake and subsequent withdrawal exert many effects on chemical processes in the brain and other tissues by a variety of mechanisms. The nature of some effects is better understood than others. More work is therefore required to elucidate little-understood mechanisms as well as to investigate possible unrecognised actions.

Few studies have been performed in man to assess the influence of ethanol on biogenic amine metabolism. Because most of these have involved examination of urinary output of amines and their metabolites, it is difficult to ascertain whether reported changes (some of which are contradictory) reflect any specific effects on cerebral biogenic amine metabolism. Detailed, more specific investigations are therefore required to elucidate any likely effects of acute and chronic ethanol consumption and subsequent withdrawal. It is also important to emphasise that animal studies have

Figure 3.4: Effects of Chronic Ethanol Administration and Subsequent Withdrawal on Tryptophan Metabolism and Disposition in the Rat

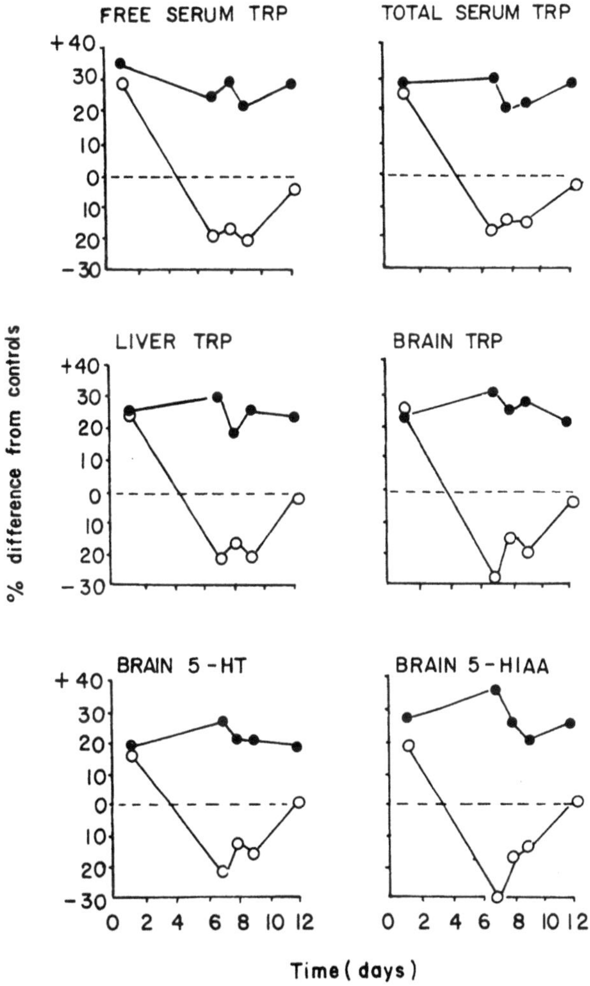

Note: Ethanol was administered in drinking water for 3 weeks to male Wistar rats. Thereafter, some rats continued to receive the drug for up to 12 days more (solid circles), whereas others were withdrawn for comparative periods (open circles). The changes observed in both chronically ethanol-treated and ethanol-withdrawn rats have been assessed by comparison with values obtained in control animals. Other details can be seen in refs 53 and 63, from which this figure is reproduced here by permission.

Figure 3.5: Effects of Chronic Ethanol Administration and Subsequent Withdrawal on Rat Liver Tryptophan Pyrrolase Activity and Serum Corticosterone Concentration

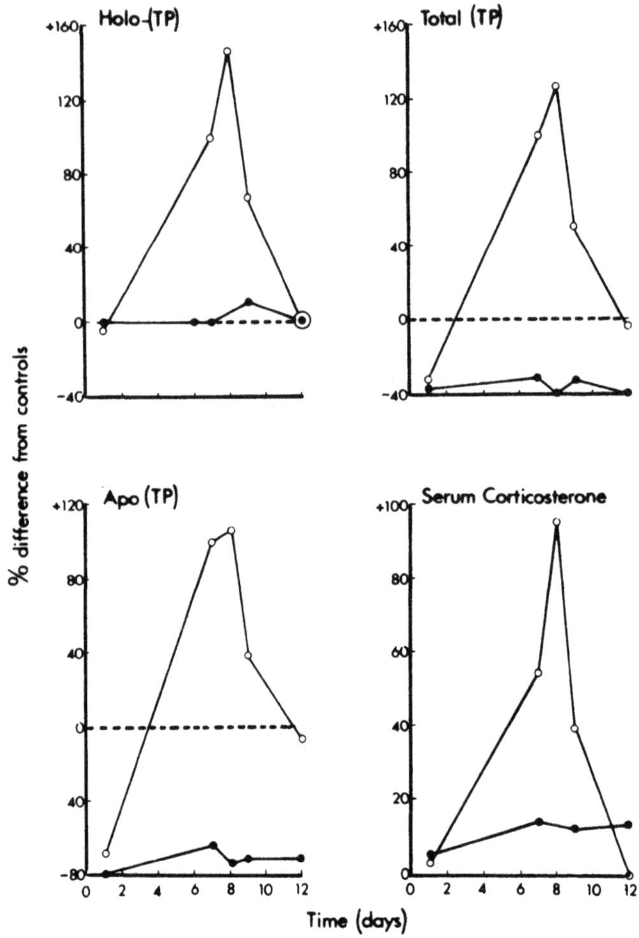

Note: All details are as described in Figure 3.4. The holo-tryptophan pyrrolase activity is that obtained in the absence, whereas the total activity is that observed in the presence, of added haematin. The activity of the apoenzyme (the haem-free predominant form in rat and human liver) is calculated by difference. This figure is reproduced here from ref. 63 by permission.

shown how cerebral biogenic amine metabolism can be influenced by very small doses of ethanol. The possibility that intake of very small amounts of alcoholic beverages (as in social or even occasional drinkers) affects biogenic amine metabolism and behaviour should not be overlooked. As the above changes in biogenic amine metabolism caused by very small doses of ethanol are associated with correspondingly small alterations in availability of the precursor amino acids, it is to be expected that behaviour associated with changes in biogenic amines could be influenced by dietary conditions or states.

The most important question in this area is whether the alcohol-induced changes in brain chemicals and processes thought to be associated with behaviour exhibit any cause-and-effect relationship with aggression. The available knowledge of the changes reviewed in this chapter is not matched by sufficient information on alcohol-induced aggressive behaviour. A few predictions could, however, be made in the light of earlier statements concerning the relationship between aggression and brain chemicals, at least in experimental animals such as the rat. Aggression may be evident later after acute intake of an intoxicating quantity or dose of ethanol and during alcohol withdrawal, because these are the time intervals at which there are decreases in brain 5-HT, GABA and catecholamines and an increase in AcCh. It must, however, be admitted that very little work has been done to address the above question of cause-and-effect or even to examine, characterise and quantify the nature and mechanism(s) of the alcohol-induced aggression, and it is therefore evident that the answers to these questions must await the outcome of extensive behavioural and biochemical investigations in man and experimental animals.

Acknowledgements

Reviewed work from this laboratory has been performed with the co-operation of many colleagues and the support of the Welsh Office, the British Medical Research Council and the British Medical Council on Alcoholism. I am grateful to Miss O. Matheson for the preparation of this typescript.

References

1. Sandler, M. in *Psychopharmacology of Aggression*, New York: Raven Press, 1979.

2. Valzelli, L. in *Psychobiology of Aggression and Violence*, New York: Raven Press, 1981.

3. Brain, P. 'Alcohol and aggression: some notes on the presumed relationship between the physiological and behavioural correlates of man's oldest drug', *British Journal on Alcohol and Alcoholism*, 1982, *17*, pp. 39-45.

4. Alkana, R.L. and Malcolm, R.D. 'Comparison of the effects of acute alcohol intoxication on behaviour in humans and other animals' in *Animal Models in Alcohol Research* (eds Eriksson, K., Sinclair, J.D. and Kiianmaa, K.), London: Academic Press, 1980, pp. 193-269.

5. Hawkins, R.D. and Kalant, H. 'The metabolism of ethanol and its metabolic effects', *Pharmacological Reviews*, 1972, *24*, pp. 67-157.

6. Badawy, A.A.-B. 'The metabolism of alcohol', *Clinics in Endocrinology and Metabolism*, 1978, *7*, pp. 247-71.

7. Majchrowicz, E. and Noble, E.P. (eds) in *Biochemistry and Pharmacology of Ethanol, vol. 1*, New York: Plenum Press, 1979.

8. Thurman, R.G. and Hoffman, P.L. (eds) in *Pharmacology, Biochemistry and Behavior*, 1983, *18, Suppl. 1.*

9. Kinard, F.W., Nelson, G.H. and Hay, M.G. 'Catalase activity and ethanol metabolism in the rat', *Proceedings of the Society of Experimental Biology and Medicine*, 1956, *92*, pp. 772-3.

10. Smith, M.E. 'Interrelations in ethanol and methanol metabolism', *Journal of Pharmacology and Experimental Therapeutics*, 1961, *134*, pp. 233-7.

11. Goodman, J.I. and Tephly, T.R. 'The role of hepatic microbody and soluble oxidase in the peroxidation of methanol in the rat and monkey', *Molecular Pharmacology*, 1968, *4*, pp. 492-501.

12. Boveris, A.G., Oshino, N. and Chance, B. 'The cellular production of hydrogen peroxide', *Biochemical Journal*, 1972, *128*, pp. 617-30.

13. Lieber, C.S. and DeCarli, L.M. 'The role of the hepatic microsomal ethanol oxidizing system (MEOS) for ethanol metabolism *in vivo*', *Journal of Pharmacology and Experimental Therapeutics*, 1972, *181*, pp. 279-87.

14. Lundquist, F. 'Enzymatic pathways of ethanol metabolism' in *International Encyclopedia of Alcohol and Alcoholism, Section 20, vol. 1* (ed. Trémolières, J.), Oxford: Pergamon Press, 1970, pp. 95-116.

15. Ribiere, C., Sinaceur, J., Nordmann, J. and Nordmann, R. 'Liver superoxide dismutases and catalase during ethanol inhalation and withdrawal', *Pharmacology, Biochemistry and Behavior*, 1983, *18, Suppl. 1*, pp. 263-6.

16. Badawy, A.A.-B. 'MEOS in alcohol metabolism', *British Journal on Alcohol and Alcoholism*, 1978, *12*, pp. 146-9.

17. Lieber, C.S. 'Microsomal ethanol oxidizing system (MEOS): interaction with ethanol, drugs and carcinogens', *Pharmacology, Biochemistry and Behavior*, 1983, *18, Suppl. 1*, pp. 181-7.

18. Winston, G.W. and Cederbaum, A.I. 'Evidence for two ethanol oxidizing pathways in reconstituted mixed-function oxidase systems' *Pharmacology, Biochemistry and Behavior*, 1983, *18, Suppl. 1*, pp. 189-94.

19. Shigeta, Y., Nomura, F., Leo, M.A., Iida, S., Felder, M.R. and Lieber, C.S. 'Alcohol dehydrogenase (ADH) independent ethanol metabolism in Deermice lacking ADH', *Pharmacology, Biochemistry and Behavior*, 1983, *18, Suppl. 1*, pp. 195-9.

20. Vind, C. and Grunnet, N. 'Interaction of cytoplasmic dehydrogenases:

quantitation of pathways of ethanol metabolism', *Pharmacology, Biochemistry and Behavior*, 1983, *18*, *Suppl. 1*, pp. 209-13.

21. Cornell, N.W. 'Properties of alcohol dehydrogenase and ethanol oxidation *in vivo* and in hepatocytes', *Pharmacology, Biochemistry and Behavior*, 1983, *18*, *Suppl. 1*, pp. 215-21.

22. Bosron, W.F., Crabb, D.W. and Li, T.-K. 'Relationship between kinetics of liver alcohol dehydrogenase and alcohol metabolism', *Pharmacology, Biochemistry and Behavior*, 1983, *18*, *Suppl. 1*, pp. 223-7.

23. Larsen, J.A., 'Extrahepatic metabolism of ethanol in man', *Nature (London)*, 1959, *184*, p. 1236.

24. Krebs, H.A., Freedland, R.A., Hems, R. and Stubbs, M. 'Inhibition of hepatic gluconeogenesis by ethanol', *Biochemical Journal*, 1969, *112*, pp. 117-24.

25. Raskin, N.H. and Sokoloff, L. 'Alcohol dehydrogenase activity in rat brain and liver', *Journal of Neurochemistry*, 1970, *17*, pp. 1677-87.

26. von Wartburg, J.P., Papenberg, J. and Albi, H. 'An atypical human alcohol dehydrogenase', *Canadian Journal of Biochemistry*, 1965, *43*, pp. 889-98.

27. Wolff, P.H. 'Ethnic differences in alcohol sensitivity', *Science*, 1972, *275*, pp. 449-50.

28. Ricciardi, B.R., Saunders, J.B., Williams, R. and Hopkinson, D.A. 'Hepatic ADH and ALDH isoenzymes in different racial groups and in chronic alcoholism', *Pharmacology, Biochemistry and Behavior*, 1983, *18*, *Suppl. 1*, pp. 61-5.

29. Pringsheim, J. 'Chemische Untersuchwegen uber das Wesen der Alkoholtoleranz', *Biochemische Zeitschrift*, 1908, *12*, pp. 143-92.

30. Cronholm, T. 'NAD^+-dependent ethanol oxidation: redox effects and rate limitation', *Pharmacology, Biochemistry and Behavior*, 1983, *18*, *Suppl. 1*, pp. 229-32.

31. Alkana, R.L. and Noble, E.P. 'Amethystic agents: reversal of acute ethanol intoxication in humans' in *Biochemistry and Pharmacology of Ethanol*, *vol. 2* (eds Majchrowicz, E. and Noble, E.P.), New York: Plenum Press, 1979, pp. 349-74.

32. Badawy, A.A.-B. and Evans, M. 'The mechanism of the antagonism by naloxone of acute alcohol intoxication', *British Journal of Pharmacology*, 1981, *74*, pp. 514-16.

33. Krebs, H.A. 'The effects of ethanol on the metabolic activities of the liver', *Advances in Enzyme Regulation*, 1968, *6*, pp. 467-80.

34. Marks, V. 'Alcohol and carbohydrate metabolism', *Clinics in Endocrinology and Metabolism*, 1978, *7*, pp. 333-49.

35. Davis, V., Brown, H., Huff, J.A. and Cashaw, J.L. 'The alteration of serotonin metabolism to 5-hydroxytryptophol by ethanol ingestion in man', *Journal of Laboratory and Clinical Medicine*, 1967, *69*, pp. 132-40.

36. Davis, V., Brown, H., Huff, J.A. and Cashaw, J.L. 'Ethanol-induced alterations of norepinephrine metabolism in man', *Journal of Laboratory and Clinical Medicine*, 1967, *69*, pp. 787-99.

37. Wright, J. 'Endocrine effects of alcohol', *Clinics in Endocrinology and Metabolism*, 1978, *7*, pp. 351-67.

38. Kakihana, R. and Butte, J.C. 'Ethanol and endocrine function' in *Biochemistry and Pharmacology of Ethanol, vol. 2* (eds Majchrowicz, E. and Noble, E.P.), New York: Plenum Press, 1979, pp. 147-64.

39. Välimäki, M. and Ylikahri, R. 'The effect of alcohol on male and female sexual function', *Alcohol and Alcoholism*, 1983, *18*, pp. 313-20.

40. Eichelman, B. 'Role of biogenic amines in aggressive behavior' in *Psychopharmacology of Aggression* (ed. Sandler, M.), 1979, New York: Raven Press, pp. 61-93.

41. Hunt, W.A. and Majchrowicz, E. 'Alterations in neurotransmitter function

after acute and chronic treatment with ethanol' in *Biochemistry and Pharmacology of Ethanol, vol. 2* (eds Majchrowicz, E. and Noble, E.P.), New York: Plenum Press, 1979, pp. 167-85.

42. Ticku, M.K., Burch, T.P. and Davis, W.C. 'The interactions of ethanol with the benzodiazepine-GABA receptor-ionophore complex', *Pharmacology, Biochemistry and Behavior*, 1983, *18, Suppl. 1*, pp. 15-18.

43. Simler, S., Kempf, E., Puglisi-Allegra, S., Ciesielski, L. and Mandel, P. 'γ-aminobutyric acid and serotonin in brain areas of isolated aggressive or non-aggressive inbred strains of mice', *Journal of Neurochemistry*, 1983, *41, Suppl. 1*, p. S105.

44. Massarelli, R. 'Effects of ethanol on the cholinergic system' in *Biochemistry and Pharmacology of Ethanol, vol. 2* (eds Majchrowicz, E. and Noble, E.P.), New York: Plenum Press, 1979, pp. 223-40.

45. Wurtman, R.J. and Fernstrom, J.D. 'Control of brain monoamine synthesis by diets and plasma amino acids', *American Journal of Clinical Nutrition*, 1975, *28*, pp. 638-47.

46. Carlsson, A. and Lindqvist, M. 'Dependence of 5-HT and catecholamine synthesis on concentrations of precursor amino-acids in rat brain', *Naunyn-Schmiedeberg's Archives für Pharmakologie*, 1978, *303*, pp. 157-64.

47. Badawy, A.A.-B. and Williams, D.L. 'Enhancement of rat brain catecholamine synthesis by administration of small doses of tyrosine and evidence for substrate inhibition of tyrosine hydroxylase activity by large doses of the amino acid', *Biochemical Journal*, 1982, *206*, pp. 165-8.

48. Badawy, A.A.-B., Williams, D.L. and Evans, M. 'Role of tyrosine in the acute effects of ethanol on rat brain catecholamine synthesis', *Pharmacology, Biochemistry and Behavior*, 1983, *18, Suppl. 1*, pp. 389-96.

49. Badawy, A.A.-B., Williams, D.L., Snape, B.M. and Evans, M. 'Brain tyrosine aminotransferase: identity and possible role in the regulation of catecholamine synthesis', *Biochemical Journal*, 1982, *204*, pp. 622-4.

50. Badawy, A.A.-B., Snape, B.M. and Evans, M. 'Biphasic effect of acute ethanol administration on rat liver tyrosine-2-oxoglutarate aminotransferase activity', *Biochemical Journal*, 1980, *186*, pp. 755-61.

51. Badawy, A.A.-B., Snape, B.M. and Evans, M. 'Biphasic enhancement of rat brain tyrosine aminotransferase activity by acute ethanol administration', *Substance and Alcohol Actions/Misuse*, 1980, *1*, pp. 517-26.

52. Badawy, A.A.-B. and Evans, M. 'The acute effects of ethanol on liver and brain tryptophan metabolism', *Advances in Experimental Medicine and Biology*, 1977, *85A*, pp. 559-69.

53. Badawy, A.A.-B., Punjani, N.F. and Evans, M. 'The effects of ethanol on rat liver and brain tryptophan metabolism', *Substance and Alcohol Actions/Misuse*, 1980, *1*, pp. 507-15.

54. Badawy, A.A.-B. 'Hepatic involvement in the effects of alcohol on brain serotonin synthesis', *British Journal on Alcohol and Alcoholism*, 1981, *16*, pp. 161-3.

55. Curzon, G. and Knott, P.J. 'Effects on plasma and brain tryptophan in the rat of drugs and hormones that influence the concentration of unesterified fatty acid in the plasma', *British Journal of Pharmacology*, 1974, *50*, pp. 197-204.

56. Fernstrom, J.D. and Wurtman, R.J. 'Brain serotonin content. Physiological regulation by plasma neutral amino acids', *Science*, 1972, *178*, pp. 414-16.

57. Badawy, A.A.-B., Punjani, N.F. and Evans, M. 'The role of liver tryptophan pyrrolase in the opposite effects of chronic administration and subsequent withdrawal of drugs of dependence on rat brain tryptophan metabolism', *Biochemical Journal*, 1981, *196*, pp. 161-70.

58. Young, S.N. 'Mechanism of the decline in rat brain 5-hydroxytryptamine

after induction of liver tryptophan pyrrolase by hydrocortisone: roles of tryptophan catabolism and kynurenine synthesis', *British Journal of Pharmacology*, 1981, *74*, pp. 695-700.

59. Badawy, A.A.-B. and Evans, M. 'The role of free serum tryptophan in the biphasic effect of acute ethanol administration on the concentrations of rat brain tryptophan, 5-hydroxytryptamine and 5-hydroxyindol-3-yl acetic acid', *Biochemical Journal*, 1976, *160*, pp. 315-24.

60. Badawy, A.A.-B., Punjani, N.F. and Evans, M. 'Unsuitability of control sucrose or glucose in studies of the effects of chronic ethanol administration on brain 5-hydroxytryptamine metabolism', *Journal of Pharmacological Methods*, 1980, *3*, pp. 167-71.

61. Badawy, A.A.-B., Punjani, N.F. and Evans, M. 'Enhancement of rat brain tryptophan metabolism by chronic ethanol administration and possible involvement of decreased liver tryptophan pyrrolase activity', *Biochemical Journal*, 1979, *178*, pp. 575-80.

62. Punjani, N.F., Badawy, A.A.-B. and Evans, M. 'Prevention by pyrazole of the effects of chronic ethanol administration on the redox states of the hepatic nicotinamide-adenine dinucleotide (phosphate) couples and on liver and brain tryptophan metabolism in the rat', *Biochemical Journal*, 1979, *184*, pp. 165-8.

63. Badawy, A.A.-B., Punjani, N.F., Evans, C.M. and Evans, M. 'Inhibition of rat brain tryptophan metabolism by ethanol withdrawal and possible involvement of the enhanced liver tryptophan pyrrolase activity', *Biochemical Journal*, 1980, *192*, 449-55.

64. Badawy, A.A.-B. and Evans, M. 'Tryptophan pyrrolase in ethanol administration and withdrawal', *Advances in Experimental Medicine and Biology*, 1973, *35*, 105-23.

65. Badawy, A.A.-B. and Evans, M. 'The effects of ethanol on tryptophan pyrrolase activity and their comparison with those of phenobarbitone and morphine', *Advances in Experimental Medicine and Biology*, 1975, *59*, 229-51.

4 A CRITICAL EVALUATION OF CLAIMED RELATIONSHIPS BETWEEN ALCOHOL INTAKE AND AGGRESSION IN INFRA-HUMAN ANIMALS

Michael S. Berry and *Robert Smoothy*

'No more alcohol for me,' said Buffy. 'Look what it does to the common earthworm'. 'But you're not a common earthworm,' I said, putting my finger on the flaw in his argument right away.'
P.G. Wodehouse, "*Summer Lightning*", 1929

Introduction

Alcohol exerts a variety of physiological effects on the nervous system[1] resulting in a wide range of behavioural changes, among which an increase in 'aggression' is often claimed to be prominent. The enormous problems of determining the relationship between alcohol and aggression in humans are discussed by Evans and Coid elsewhere in this volume. Animal studies, with their reduced methodological and ethical problems, might be expected to provide a clearer picture of the association between alcohol and aggression. The subjects are said to have less complex social structures and nervous systems than humans, facilitating the examination of the causes, and the effects of drugs on aggression.[2] They have failed, however, to produce the anticipated clear-cut results. Some workers have claimed that ethanol stimulates aggression in animals, whereas others have found no effect or a suppression of these activities. A multitude of methodological variations between available studies seem likely to account for these discrepancies: alcohol's behavioural correlates have been assessed in diverse situations, at a variety of doses or concentrations, using different routes of administration and at a variety of times after administration. Other variables, such as the choice of testing arena, and the species, strain, sex, age and social status of subjects used, may also substantially affect the results obtained.

This chapter seeks to clarify the seemingly diverse and often conflicting results of experiments on alcohol and infra-human aggression. It specifically examines the frequent claim that alcohol exerts a biphasic effect on aggression, increasing it at low doses and decreasing it at higher doses.

Alcohol and Aggression in Fish

The Siamese fighting fish (*Betta splendens*) and the Convict cichlid (*Cichlasoma nigrofasciatum*) have been much used in research on alcohol and aggression. They are considered useful because they are reliably aggressive in defence of a territory, their responses tend to be stereotyped,[3] and blood alcohol can be maintained at steady concentrations by controlling the amount of alcohol in the aquarium water.[4,5,6,] In a typical study on male *B. splendens*, a low concentration of alcohol (285mg per cent) was added to the tank water for a period of 6 hours.[3] Attack was elicited by presenting the resident with a live male conspecific held in a glass box and measuring the number of approaches made towards this 'target' fish. Such approaches were punished by means of electric shocks (electrodes were placed in front of the 'target') in an attempt to determine whether alcohol facilitated aggression by disinhibition (i.e. reducing 'fear' of the consequences). This appeared to be the case, as fish receiving alcohol required three times the number of shocks to suppress approach (although the possibility that alcohol acts as an analgesic or pain reliever cannot be ruled out). Subsequent experiments in which the aggressive response was measured without punishment, also revealed facilitation by the same dose of alcohol. This suggests that the previous results were not simply due to analgesia, and that alcohol stimulated aggression directly, as there was no obvious inhibitory factor.[3,7] Here, aggression was assessed by the cumulative time that the gill cover was lowered in response to a mirror image of the fish: this is an all-or-none response and is therefore easily quantified.[8,9] The use of a mirror image in aggression tests has been criticised,[4] however, since it may provide an unnatural stimulus for attack: *Bettas* generally face each other at right angles in agonistic encounters.[10] A somewhat high alcohol concentration of 650mg per cent decreased such responding,[3] and it was suggested that alcohol has a biphasic action (potentiating aggression at lower and decreasing it at higher doses).

A biphasic response to alcohol has also been reported in studies on *C. nigrofasciatum*, where alcohol was again added directly to the aquarium water.[4,11,12] Residents were presented with a live, male conspecific confined in a glass tube, and a variety of aggressive responses (including biting and displaying frequencies) were recorded. Interestingly, the dose suppressing aggression in *C. nigrofasciatum* was very similar to that potentiating this response in *Betta*, suggesting that there may be marked species differences in sensitivity to the effects of the same dose of alcohol. Unfortunately, it cannot be ascertained whether this differential sensitivity is the result of the two species attaining different blood-alcohol levels, since this measurement was only determined for *C. nigrofasciatum*. Failure of the fish to emerge from its refuge or to engage in aggressive behaviour was regarded as a sign of 'timidity', and this progressively increased with elevations of alcohol dose.

Subsequent research has assessed the effects of alcohol on both initiation and habituation (i.e. the gradual reduction with time) of aggression in *C. nigrofasciatum*, tested as above over a 30-min period.[13] Display and biting frequencies showed biphasic responses to alcohol, being potentiated at the low dose (150mg per cent) and suppressed at the high dose (300mg per cent). Over the test, control fish showed a progressive decrease in displaying and an increase in biting. Threat, therefore, initially preceded the appearance of 'violent' behaviour, which the authors suggested provided a mechanism where disputes could be settled by threat alone. Behavioural topographies in fish treated with alcohol were, however, very different. At the low dose, fish showed short displays with high rates of biting and relatively little threat, which was interpreted as a tendency for the fish to attack without warning. At the high dose, the display frequency was reduced, but was actually of longer duration than in controls — if long-duration threat displays characterise the early stages in aggressive encounters, high alcohol dosage appears to retard the progression of the sequence. The results suggest that alcohol has profound quantitative and qualitative effects on the elicitation and habituation of social conflict aggression in Convict cichlids, and the biphasic response shows that alcohol does not act as a simple inhibitor of aggression in this situation.[13]

These biphasic effects of alcohol on Convict cichlids were used in an attempt to determine the mechanisms underlying the 'prior residence effect'[14] (i.e. the dominance advantage of a territorial resident over an intruder[15,16]). Alcohol (up to 350mg per cent) was given to either the resident fish or an intruder (never to both) in direct encounters, with both fish freely interacting. Changes in dominance (recorded as biting, butting and showing of frontal or lateral displays[17,18,19]) only occurred as a result of drugging the resident: there was no difference between controls and a low dose (150mg per cent), but fish given doses of 200 and 350mg per cent failed to show a significant prior residence effect. Alcohol therefore decreased aggression at doses as low as 200mg per cent in this free-interaction social conflict situation, and the absence of a low-dose potentiation is in marked contrast to earlier studies on these fish.

Humans rarely drink pure ethanol, preferring various alcoholic beverages containing many different additional compounds known as congeners; including organic acids, aldehydes and esters which lend the flavour, colour and characteristic properties to these liquids.[20,21] Attempts to determine possible effects of congeners and beverage alcohols on aggression have been carried out in fish.[7,12,22] Early work using *B. splendens* showed that exposure to pure ethanol solution increased responding towards a mirror image,[7] but both bourbon and a solution of bourbon congeners reduced responding. This suggests that (a) ethanol is not the only psychoactive component of alcoholic beverages; and (b) these bourbon congeners may have an inhibitory effect that counteracts the aggression-enhancing effect of ethanol alone. In *C. nigrofasciatum* neither very low doses of pure ethanol (100mg per cent) nor solutions of bourbon or brandy diluted to produce the same ethanol concentrations had any marked effect on aggression.[22] A comparable solution of rum, however, suppressed aggressive responses directed towards a 'target' fish in a glass tube. A solution of acetaldehyde (a major congener) decreased display frequency and biting frequency in this species. The suppression of aggression by rum was not, however, entirely due to its acetaldehyde content, and it was concluded that other components of this beverage contributed to the observed inhibition. Thus, different alcoholic beverages (even with the same alcohol content) can have variable effects on aggressive responding, presumably as a result of variations in their congener content. The effects of congeners on aggression are currently limited to fish studies, but results indicate that such investigations could be profitably extended to other animals.

These studies on social conflict in fish suggest that alcohol has a biphasic effect on aggression, potentiating responses at low doses and suppressing them at high doses, although these doses vary for different species. In the single study which more naturalistically allowed the animals to freely interact, however, there was *no* potentiation of aggression even at low doses.[14] The dose range that potentiates social conflict aggression appears to be extremely narrow: in *C. nigrofasciatum*, for example, increases in aggression were only found at 150 to 180mg per cent (average blood-alcohol levels of 97.5 to 117mg per cent respectively); suppression occurred at 200mg per cent and above;[4,13,14] whilst doses below 150mg per cent[14,22] had no effect. Potentiation of aggression by a low and narrow range of doses is also characteristic of other groups of animals (see later). It has been suggested that these biphasic effects of alcohol in fish[4] are analagous to the alcohol-aggression associations claimed in humans, e.g. in people arrested during or immediately after a felony.[23] However, the majority had urine-alcohol concentrations between 100 and 300mg per cent, obviously a much wider range than in fish.

One problem associated with fish studies is that the drug is administered by immersing the test animal directly in the alcohol solution, making it impossible to rule out a peripheral influence of alcohol, e.g. as a painful or irritant stimulus.[24,25] Other problems concern the failure to measure the blood-alcohol concentration (BAC) in some studies, preventing meaningful comparisons; the rate of alcohol uptake is species specific and it is hazardous to base assumptions about BACs in one species from uptake data in another.[4,26] For *C. nigrofasciatum*, the final BAC averaged 65 per cent of the tank ethanol concentration at both low and high doses, levels that were reached 5-6 hours after immersion;[4] in contrast, levels in the goldfish (*Crassius auratus*) reach 85 per cent after a similar length of time.[6]

Data for fish studies are summarised in Table 4.1.

Alcohol and Aggression in Amphibians

The only study on alcohol and amphibian 'aggression' concerns prey-catching habituation in Leopard frogs (*Rana pipiens*).[27] It is included because predation has been considered as a form of aggression, although it is clearly distinct from competitive or defensive forms of attack.[28] Leopard frogs were placed for 2-5 hours in a 400mg per cent solution of alcohol, allowing its absorp-

Table 4.1: Effect of Alcohol on Aggression in Fish

Authors	Animal	Age	Arena	Behavioural test	Drug recipient	Ethanol dose (mg/100ml)	Effect on aggression
3	Siamese fighting fish, *Betta splendens*			Approaches towards target fish, punished by electric shocks	Test animal	285	↑
				Response to mirror image	Test animal	285	↑
						650	↓
7	Siamese fighting fish, *B. splendens*			Response to mirror image	Test animal	285 (as ethanol)	↑
						285 (as bourbon)	↓
4,11	Convict cichlid, *Cichlasoma nigrofasciatum*	Adult	Home	Resident's response to live male conspecific presented in a glass tube	Resident	70	—
						180	↑
						330	↓
13	Convict cichlid, *C. nigrofasciatum*	Adult	Home	Resident's response to live male conspecific presented in a glass tube	Resident	150	↑
						300	↓ (↑)
14	Convict cichlid, *C. nigrofasciatum*	Adult	Home	Resident v. intruder situation, fish freely interacting	Intruder	150, 200, 350	Intruder: — Resident: —
					Resident	150	—
						200, 350	↓
32	Convict cichlid, *C. nigrofasciatum*	Adult	Home	Resident's response to live male conspecific presented in a glass tube	Resident	100 (as ethanol)	—
						100 (as bourbon or brandy)	— (↓)
						100 (as rum)	↓ (↑)

Table 4.1: continued

Note: In all cases, individually housed male fish were immersed in an alcohol solution in the aquarium for 6 hours prior to testing. See also refs 12 and 26.
Key:
↑ – increase in aggression prevalent, but not necessarily an effect on all aspects of aggressive behaviour.
↓ – decrease in aggression prevalent, but not necessarily an effect on all aspects of aggressive behaviour.
↑ (↓) – increase in aggression prevalent, but some aspects showing indications of a decrease — such results illustrate the danger of relying on single measures of aggression rather than recording the whole behavioural repertoire.
↓ (↑) – decrease in aggression prevalent, but some aspects showing indications of an increase.
— – aggression levels unchanged.
Is – Isolated (individually housed) subjects.
Gp – group-housed subjects.
p.o – per os.
Arenas described as 'Unfamiliar' refer to any testing location other than the home cage of the subject.

tion through the skin. The animal was then placed in a vertical transparent cylinder suspended just above a rotating horizontal disc. A dummy 'worm' (a painted rod) which represented the prey object was located near the perimeter of the disc, and the frequency of orientating or snapping/striking responses made to this target was recorded. Although both the alcohol-treated and control groups showed habituation of the response, it was less obvious in the alcohol group. These effects were reproducible with 400mg per cent, but not with 300 or 500mg per cent. The results support the findings on the effects of alcohol on habituation in *C. nigrofasciatum*, particularly at higher doses, where this process was retarded.[13] Since alcohol retards habituation of this visually elicited prey-catching response, the results may reflect an alcohol-induced disinhibition within the visuomotor mechanism (probably the optic tectum).[27] The caudal thalamus is thought to inhibit the optic tectum (since lesions of the former area disinhibit prey-catching[29]). Alcohol may decrease the activity or responsiveness of the caudal thalamus, releasing units within the optic tectum from normal inhibitory modulation.

Data for this study on amphibians are summarised in Table 4.2.

Table 4.2: Effect of Alcohol on 'Aggression' in Amphibians

Authors	Animal	Age	Arena	Behavioural test	Drug recipient	Route of administration	Time after admini-stration	Ethanol dose (mg %)	Effect on aggression
27	Leopard frog *Rana pipiens*		Unfamiliar	Responses made towards artificial prey object	Test animal	Absorbed through skin	2-5 hours	400	Decreased habituation

Alcohol and Aggression in Birds

Studies on birds have concentrated on the long-term effects of alcohol administered acutely in relatively high doses. For example, White Leghorn cocks (*Gallus domesticus*) were orally given grain alcohol by mouth or an equal quantity of water orally, 30 min before exposure to six White Rock chicks.[30] Cocks were immobilised by holding the bird supine with the beak held vertically (making the bird fall into an immobile, drowsy state), and chicks were placed between the body and wings for a 30-min period. The cock was then observed over subsequent days, and its behaviour towards the chicks recorded. The alcohol-treated birds tended to develop maternal behaviour such as sheltering and defending the chicks, whilst controls only showed avoidance and aggression. Therefore alcohol, at a relatively high dose (approximately 2.3g alcohol/kg body wt) suppressed aggression. The author suggested that observed maternal behaviour was not directly dependent upon hormonal mechanisms, since alcohol has not been identified as a prolactin releaser or inhibitor of androgen (prolactin effectively stimulates maternal behaviour in the cock as it inhibits androgen secretion[31]). This study was initiated because of an old custom amongst Hungarian farmers, of transferring newly hatched chicks from the hen to a 'drunken cock', the benefits being that cocks are better than hens at defending chicks from predators, and the hens are freed for commercially desirable egg-laying. A similar study was performed on White Rock cocks and chicks.[32] Cocks were given water or high doses of grain alcohol, and then presented with chicks as before.[30] Control birds generally killed, pecked at and avoided the chicks, whereas alcohol-treated cocks sheltered, defended and clucked at chicks.

These long-term suppressions of aggression were not confirmed in studies of social conflict behaviour using highly aggressive, experienced gamecocks (*Gallus gallus*).[33] Pairs of birds were given very high doses of ethanol (about 2.6 to 7.8g/kg body wt) directly into the stomach via gastric intubation, then left together and allowed to recover. The low dose caused slight stupefaction, whilst higher doses led to 'profound depression' and anaesthesia, sometimes lasting more than six hours. Aggression was abolished during intoxication along with all other motor-behaviour, but upon recovery from the effects of alcohol there was no effect on this attribute as estimated by attack latency. This is in contrast to previous avian studies,[30,32] where long-lasting attenuation of aggressive activities was observed. Any potentiation of aggression was unlikely to be observed, due to the extremely short attack latencies. No firm conclusions are possible since only very small numbers of birds were used (in some cases, only a single pair per dose).

These few available studies on alcohol and aggression in birds allow no general conclusions to be drawn. Restricted models of aggression were used, doses of alcohol were high, blood-alcohol levels were unknown, and the effects of grain alcohol may not be the same as ethanol (due to the presence of congeners). Data for these studies are summarised in Table 4.3.

Alcohol and Aggression in Rodents

The bulk of animal experiments on alcohol and aggression have been carried out on rodents, especially laboratory mice and rats. Three broad experimental designs have been used: (1) alcohol administered to the parent, followed by observation of the offsprings' behaviour; (2) acute or chronic administration to the test animal; and (3) self-administration (i.e. drinking) of ethanol by the test animal itself.

(1) *Pre-natal Alcohol Administration*

Little work is available on the effects of acute alcohol treatment of parents on the subsequent aggressive behaviour of their offspring. Studies generally concentrate on chronic drug administration, probably because excessive drinking in humans may produce the 'foetal alcohol syndrome' (i.e. offspring with physical and mental abnormalities). Some workers report increases in subsequent aggression in rodents, whilst others have found no effect or a suppression (a similar diversity to that found when alcohol is given directly to the test animals themselves — see later).

Krsiak, Elis, Poschlova and Masek[34,35] showed that administration of ethanol to mice during pregnancy may increase their offsprings' aggressive behaviour. Alcohol was given orally to pregnant female mice for the whole of the gestation period at a moderate dose of 1g/kg/day, control females being given water.[34] After weaning and a period of housing in single-sex cages, male offspring were individually housed for five weeks, and then tested for

Table 4.3: Effect of Alcohol on Aggression in Birds

Authors	Animal	Age	Type	Behavioural test	Arena	Drug recipient	Route of administration	Time after administration	Ethanol dose (g/kg)	Effect on aggression
30	White Leghorn cocks, *Gallus domesticus*	9 months		Exposing immobilised bird to chicks and recording maternal responses		Test animal	p.o.	60 mins to 5 days	2.3 (as grain alcohol	↓
32	White Rock cocks, *Gallus domesticus*	12 months		Exposing immobilised bird to chicks and recording maternal responses		Test animal	p.o.	60 mins to 5 days	1.3, 2-6 (as grain alcohol)	↓
33	Game cocks, *Gallus gallus*	Adult	Experienced in cock fighting	Fighting in paired birds following recovery from alcohol	Unfamiliar	Both birds	Gastric intubation	Various	2.6 to 7-8	— (following recovery)

Key as for Table 4.1.

aggression in encounters with a group-housed male. There were no differences in the duration of pregnancy and number of offspring in alcohol-treated and control mice, but offspring from alcohol-treated parents showed more attack, tail-rattling and 'aggressive unrest' in response to opponents. All other aspects of social behaviour including social investigation of the partner and defensive responses were unchanged.

Increases in animal aggressivity have been associated with increased brain catecholamine activity.[36] Krsiak *et al.*[35] (using a similar procedure and alcohol dosage/administration regimen to the above study[34]) found, however, that brain catecholamine (dopamine and noradrenaline) levels were not significantly different in offspring from alcohol-treated or control parents. This does not preclude the possibility of changes in metabolism, however, as offspring of alcohol-treated rats show increased activity of tyrosine hydroxylase in the caudate nucleus, indicating increased turnover of dopamine.[37] Krsiak *et al.*[35] found significantly reduced levels of serotonin, which may also be associated with increases in aggression, (Valzelli[38] has demonstrated lower levels of serotonin in aggressive than in non-aggressive mice).

These findings are generally in agreement with various human studies; for example, many children with hyperactivity (including increased aggression) have alcoholic parents.[39] There is also evidence that the hyperactive syndrome in man involves decreased activity of the brain serotonergic system.[40] In apparent contrast, however, several other studies with rodents have revealed no increases in aggression in offspring of alcohol-treated parents; indeed, in some cases there appeared to be a marked depression. There were, however, obvious methodological differences in the various studies, including the doses of alcohol given to the mothers, and the age of offspring at testing. The studies which found subsequent decreases in aggression invariably used higher alcohol doses and exposed the offspring earlier in life.

A decrease in 'aggression' has been found using a model of predatory behaviour in two strains of mice.[41] Parent mice were housed in single-sex groups of four following weaning, and given an ethanol solution as their only source of liquid (control mice were given water). Animals were mated and pregnant females were given alcohol in their drinking water until 14 days *post partum.* Alcohol was consumed at a rate of 10-15g/kg/day at mating age, and 12-28g/kg/day during nursing (cf 1g/kg/day in the previously mentioned studies[34,35]). The responses of offspring of both sexes to a live, adult cricket (*Acheta domesticus*) were tested on two successive days (studies of the stomach contents of feral mice have shown that insects are a major dietary item[42,43]). Numbers of mice showing attack and the percentage of successful attacks were reduced in alcohol-treated mice, but only significantly so in the DBA strain (a highly inbred laboratory strain). Thus, early ethanol exposure induced chronic physiological changes (probably neural[41]) which resulted in a long-term reduction of predation.

The effects of early ethanol exposure on intermale fighting were examined in the above two strains of mice.[44] Breeding females were given ethanol solution to drink from 28 days of age up to 14 days *post partum.* Male offspring of such mice were less aggressive than counterparts from water-treated controls. A reduction in fighting was most obvious in the more highly aggressive DBA strain. Later experiments confirmed the suppression of intermale fighting in the offspring of parents consuming large quantities of alcohol.[45] As ethanol supplies calories, 'nutritional control' parents were employed in addition to water-treated controls. Nutritional controls were given an isocaloric glucose solution and their food intake matched to that of the experimental group. The offspring from these controls were similar to counterparts from water-treated controls, indicating that nutritional differences did not account for observed variations in aggression (under-nutrition usually increases aggression[46,47,48]). The weights of offspring from ethanol and nutritional control groups were identical, but significantly lower than the water control category. The authors suggest that this weight difference may be due to both ethanol and glucose inhibiting milk let-down.

Attempts have been made to determine the period at which offspring are most sensitive to alcohol.[45] Female mice were given alcohol from the 28th day of life until their pups were born, or from the day of birth of their pups and the next 14 days. Offspring given prenatal exposure to ethanol were behaviourally similar to water-treated controls. Postnatally exposed mice had increased attack latencies and showed decreased numbers of 'aggressive' periods. The postnatal period consequently seemed the more sensitive time for early ethanol effects, although there was the possibility of a dose effect since lactating mothers consumed greater quantities of alcohol. Rodents and humans are not directly comparable, however, as there is considerable postnatal maturation of the rat's brain during the first few days after birth, whereas in man, the major period of brain growth begins in mid-pregnancy.[49]

Alcohol may also cause other morphological changes such as decreasing mean pup weight and delaying onset of fur development,[50] confirming that nutritional controls are important in such studies. Even relatively low alcohol doses (1-2g/kg/day) administered chronically during pregnancy can affect litter size and weight,[51] although other studies have found no such effects even at doses as high as 8g/kg/day.[52] Data for studies on prenatal alcohol administration in rodents are summarised in Table 4.4.

(2) *Direct Alcohol Administration*

A wide variety of 'models' of aggression have been used here, including predatory, pain-induced and intermale (social conflict) aggression (the latter frequently generated by individual housing).

(i) *Predatory Attack.* Alcohol's effects have been studied on mouse-killing ('muricidal') behaviour in rats.[53] Rats were allocated to categories that killed mice, did not kill mice, or initially killed but subsequently stopped. Ethanol tested over a range of low to high doses neither induced muricide in 'non-killers', nor re-established killing in 'stopped killers'. Higher doses suppressed predation in 'killer' rats, an effect which may reflect ataxia (impairment of movement). Lower doses of alcohol had no effect on 'killer' rats. This, the only available study on predatory attack in rodents under the influence of direct alcohol administration, presents no evidence for a biphasic effect of alcohol on aggression.

(ii) *Pain-induced or Defensive Aggression.* The situation most frequently employed involves the application of unavoidable footshocks to paired animals in a confined area. Animals in this situation tend to leap, run, assume upright postures and fight each other. In rats, the 'aggression' elicited by electric shock has been described as 'self-defensive'[54,55,56] or 'irritable'[57] aggression, but such fighting may be more offensive in mice.[58] One should note that alcohol may have analgesic properties and weaken the stimulus for such aggression in treated animals.[59]

High doses of alcohol have been given to female mice 30 min before placing pairs of such animals on a grid within a glass cylinder and subjecting them to a predetermined optimal shock

Table 4.4: Effect of Pre-natally Administered Alcohol on Aggression in Offspring of Rodents

Authors	Animal	Age of offspring	Sex of offspring	Type of offspring	Behavioural test	Arena	Dose regimen	Route of administration	Ethanol dose (g/kg/day)	Effect on aggression
34	Mice	About 17 weeks	Male	Is for 5 weeks	Isolate v. group-housed male mouse, paired interaction		Throughout whole period of gestation	p.o.	1	↑
41	C57 and DBA strain mice	50-51 days	Male and female	Is for 24 hours	Animal presented with prey object: a live cricket	Home	10% v/v solution, from weaning, throughout gestation; up to 14 days *post partum*	In drinking water	10-15 at mating age; 12-28 during nursing	↓
44	C57 and DBA mice		Male		Paired interaction		10% v/v solution from weaning up to 14 days *post partum*	In drinking water	11.7-23.4(?)	↓
35	Randomly bred albino mice	15-18 weeks	Male	Is for 5 weeks	Isolate v. group-housed male mouse, paired interaction	Unfamiliar	20% w/v solution, throughout gestation	p.o.	1	↑
45	C57 and DBA mice	50-52 days	Male	Is for 22 days	Paired interactions (isolate v. isolate) within same treatment	Unfamiliar	10% v/v solution from weaning up to 14 days *post partum*	In drinking water	10-15 at mating age, 12-28 during nursing	↓
	DBA mice	50-52 days	Male	Is for 22 days	Paired interactions (isolate v. isolate) within same treatment	Unfamiliar	10% v/v solution from weaning up to day of birth of pups	In drinking water	10-15	—
							10% v/v solution from day of birth of pups to 14 days *post partum*	In drinking water	12-28	↓
50	CFW mice	3-4 and 18-24 weeks	Male and female	Gp	Paired interaction between alcohol-treated and control-treated partner of the same sex	Unfamiliar	*5% solution, 3 weeks before mating up to post-weaning. 5% solution given to offspring from weaning onwards	In drinking water	17 (on average)	—

Note: Alcohol was given exclusively to the parents of test animals except where indicated (*), where it was also given to the offspring. Key as for Table 4.1.

intensity and frequency over a 3-min period.[60] The lowest alcohol dose (1.2g/kg) had no effect, but higher doses decreased fighting duration. As decreased arousal and pronounced ataxia were evident, the effects on fighting seem non-specific.

Alcohol was intraperitoneally injected into rats at a variety of doses 15 min before testing in a shock box.[61] Ethanol-treated rats were paired with saline-injected partners, and the pair subjected to a fixed frequency of electric shocks (the shock intensity was varied for different pairs according to pre-drug estimations of the intensity required to induce fighting). Only the percentage of shocks delivered that resulted in fighting were recorded, but it is unclear whether this activity was seen in the alcohol-treated rat alone or both subjects. Some animals had to be withdrawn from the experiment as they became too weak to continue (!) and the missing data were estimated. Compared to controls a 'significant' increase at the low dose (0.6g/kg) and a decrease at the highest dose were evident. The actual data, however, revealed non-significant effects at all doses; thus the evidence for potentiation is weak. The conclusions tend to be supported, however, by an unpublished study on shock-induced aggression in rats, in which alcohol injections increased fighting cf saline-injected controls[62] and by studies on chronic alcohol administration in a tube-testing situation[63,64] (see later).

In contrast, subsequent work on shock-induced social fighting in rats has failed to demonstrate a potentiation of aggression by alcohol.[53] Low doses had no effect on aggression when given to one or both members of the pair subjected to electric shocks in a free-interaction situation, whereas higher doses tended to suppress such activities. The methodological weaknesses of the earlier cited study[61] did not apply, so the absence of a defensive aggression-elevation by alcohol appears more convincing than claims to the contrary. This may also be related to the experimental design used in the two studies (see later).

A further model of 'aggression' that may be self-defensive[28] is the tube-restraint paradigm.[65,66,67] Animals confined in a narrow tube will bite metal targets with or without the administration of electric shocks.[68] In one such study where rats were given electric shocks, low to moderate doses of alcohol given acutely 15 min before testing did not alter biting frequencies compared to saline-injected controls.[69] After two hours, however, there was a significant decrease in responding in animals given a dose as low as

0.6g/kg. Tube-restraint experiments on mice unexposed to electric shocks also show no significant potentiation of biting at low, moderate or high acute doses of alcohol in subjects tested 20 min after administration.[70,71] Animals showed a dose-related suppression of biting, with decreases in biting frequency and increases in biting latency at 1.0 and 2.0g/kg. Low doses (0.25 and 0.5g/kg)[72] had no such effects.

Chronic administration of alcohol to rats tested in a shock-induced/tube-restraint situation suggest a biphasic response; doses of 1.97 and 3.9g/kg/day tend to increase biting frequencies whilst a higher dose of 5.9g/kg/day suppresses this activity.[63,64] The potentiation is in contrast to results on acute administration in this situation.[64,69] The results parallel the earlier cited findings of Weitz,[61] which was also, in effect, a chronic study, since a repeated-measures design was employed. It may also explain the increased aggression reported by some groups and the lack of potentiation recorded by others,[53,70,71] since all the latter used acute administration. Thus, chronic alcohol administration seems to potentiate aggression in such situations, whereas acute treatment does not produce this effect. High doses suppress aggression irrespective of experimental design.

Data for these studies are summarised in Table 4.5.

(iii) *Intermale or Social-conflict Aggression.* Drug effects on behaviour in social-conflict situations are commonly assessed using intermale encounters in which paired animals interact freely in the absence of obviously noxious stimuli. Baseline levels of aggressiveness can be increased by individually housing one (or both) members of the pair for varying periods. The aggression observed in these situations differs from that seen in pain-induced studies since it is generally claimed to be (a) competitive and (b) somewhat ritualised, involving injury-limiting strategies.[28]

Multiple behavioural indices in these free-interaction situations may be superior to reliance solely on aggression measures, in that selective drug effects are more easily distinguished.[73] For example, does alcohol reduce all upright postures (perhaps non-specifically) or does it only affect those upright postures associated with particular motivations (e.g. upright offensive cf non-social rearing)? Use of ethologically inspired techniques reveals that alcohol may specifically decrease elements of aggressive behaviour in isolated mice in encounters with group-housed male mice, whilst leaving

Table 4.5: Effect of Alcohol Administration on Aggression in Rodents

Authors	Animal	Age	Type	Behavioural test	Arena	Drug recipient	Time after administration (min)	Route of administration	Ethanol dose (g/kg)	Effect on aggression
60	Swiss-Webster mice*	6 weeks		Shock-induced fighting	Unfamiliar	Test animal	30	p.o.	1.2, 2.4, 4.7.	↓
74	Swiss mice		Is	Isolate v. group-housed male mouse		Opponent		p.o.	0.64, 1.6	Isolate: —
									4.0	Isolate: ↓
73	Mice		Is	Isolate v. group-housed male		Test animal		p.o.,	1.6	↓
						Opponent		p.o.		Isolate: ↓
						Both		p.o.	1.6	Isolate: ↓
81	LACA mice	13 weeks	Is for 1 week	Isolate v. isolated male	Home cage	Test animal**			0.5**	↑
77, 78	Wistar rats		Is for 24 hours; previously pair-housed	Resident v. removed partner (re-introduced to cage)	Home cage of pair	Test animal (separated partner)	30	p.o.	1.2, 3.0	↓
						Opponent (separated partner)	30	p.o.	1.2	Resident: —
									3.0	Resident: ↓
61	Hooded rats	~ 240 days	Is for 216 days	Shock-induced fighting, isolate v. isolate	Unfamiliar	Test animal	15	i.p.	0.6	(↑)
									1.2, 1.8	—
82	Random-bred albino mice		Is for 3-6 weeks (a) 'Aggressive'	Isolate v. group-housed male mouse	Unfamiliar	Test animal	30	p.o.	0.4	
									0.8, 1.6, 2.4.	↓
			(b) 'Sociable'	Isolate v. group-housed male	Unfamiliar	Test animal	30	p.o.	0.4, 0.8, 1.6, 2.4	—
			(c) 'Timid'	Isolate v. group-housed male	Unfamiliar	Test animal	30	p.o.	0.4	—
									0.8	↑
									1.6, 2.4	—

Table 4.5 continued

85	Sprague-Dawley rats		Is (a) Dominant	Withholding food reward-dominant v. subordinate opponent	Unfamiliar	Test animal	10	i.p.	0.5	↑
									1.0	—
			(b) Subordinate	Withholding food reward-subordinate v. dominant opponent	Unfamiliar	Test animal	10	i.p.	0.5, 1.0, 1.5	—
			(c) Naïve	Withholding food reward-naïve v. dominant opponent	Unfamiliar	Test animal	10	i.p.	1.0, 1.5	—
91	Swiss-Webster mice	60-80 days	Is for 3 days	Isolate v. isolate	Home cage	Both animals	15-795	i.p.	0.4, 1.2	↓
25	TA and TNA mice	2-6 months	Is for 1-5 months	Isolate v. standard opponent	Home cage	Test animal	15	i.p.	1.0	—
	TA mice	10-11 months	Is for 9-10 months	Isolate v standard opponent	Home cage	Test animal	20	i.p.	1.0, 1.5	(↑)
							50	i.p.	1.0, 1.5	—
	TA and TNA mice	6-7 months	Is for 5-6 months	Isolate v. standard opponent	Home cage	Test animal	20	i.p.	1.0, 1.5	—
24	TA mice	3 months	Is for 3 weeks	Isolate v. standard opponent		Test animal	15	i.p.	1.5	—
86	Swiss-Webster mice	10-12 weeks	Pair housed with female	Reproductively experienced male v. group housed male	Home cage	Test animal	30	p.o.	0.3, 0.6, 1.2.	—
					Unfamiliar	Test animal	30	p.o.	0.3,	↑
									0.6	—
									1.2	↓

69	Albino-rats	180 days	Is	Shock induced, tube-restraint 'aggression'	Unfamiliar	Test animal	15	i.p.	0.6, 1.2	—
	Sprague-Dawley rats	180 days	Is	Shock induced, tube-restraint 'aggression'	Unfamiliar	Test animal	120	i.p.	0.6	↓
95	Swiss mice	55-59 days	Is for 14 days	Isolate v. standard opponent	Home cage	Test animal	20	i.p.	0.1, 0.5, 1.0	↓
98, 99	Swiss mice	55-65 days	Is for 14-16 days. 'Aggressively rated individuals'	Isolate v. standard opponent	Home cage	Test animal	20	i.p.	0.5, 1.0, 2.0	↓
53	Sprague-Dawley rats		Gp	Shock-induced fighting, group-housed v. group-housed	Unfamiliar	Both animals	25	i.p.	0.25, 0.5, 1.0	—
						Test animals	25	i.p.	0.25, 0.5, 1.0, 1.5, 2.0.	— (↓)
53	Sprague-Dawley rats†		Is (a) killer-rats	'Muricidal' attack by rat on mouse	Home cage	Test animal	5, 30, 60, 120	i.p.	0.25, 0.5, 1.0	—
									1.5, 2.0	↓
			(b) Non-killers and stopped killers	'Muricidal' attack by rat on mouse	Home cage	Test animal	0-1200	i.p.	0.25, 0.5, 1.0, 1.5, 2.0	—
88	Swiss mice	55-65 days	Is for 14 dys	Isolate v. female intruder	Home cage	Test animal	20	i.p.	0.5	—
									1.0, 2.0	↓
76	Swiss-Webster Mice	Adult	Pair housed with female	Reproductively experienced male v. group housed male	Home	Intruder	15	p.o.	0.3, 1.0, 1.7	Resident: —
									3.0	Resident: ↑
	Long-Evans rats	Adult	Pair housed with female	Reproductively experienced male v. isolated male	Home	Intruder	15	p.o.	0.1, 0.3, 0.6, 1.0	Resident: —
									1.7	Resident: ↑

Table 4.5 continued

75	Mice		Pair housed with female	Reproductively experienced male v intruder male	Home	Resident		p.o.	0.5, 1.0	↑
									2.0	↓
						Intruder		p.o.	0.5	Resident: —
									1.0, 2.0	Resident: ↑
63	Albino rats	180 days	Is	Shock-induced, tube-restraint 'aggression'	Unfamiliar	Test animal	15	i.p.	1.97, 3.9 for 15 days	↑
									5.9 for 15 days	↓
64	Albino rats	120 days	Is	Shock-induced, tube-restraint 'aggression'	Unfamiliar	Test animal	15	i.p.	1.97	↓
									1.97 for 15 days	↑
70, 72	Swiss mice	65-70 days	Gp	Tube-restraint target-biting	Unfamiliar	Test animal	20	i.p.	0.25, 0.5	—
									1.0, 2.0	↓
			Is for 16 days	Tube-restraint target-biting	Unfamiliar	Test animal	20	i.p.	0.5, 1.0	—
									2.0	↓
		120-130 days	Gp experienced in tube test situation	Tube restraint target-biting	Unfamiliar	Test animal	20	i.p.	0.5	—
									1.0, 2.0	↓
			Is for 14 days, experienced in test tube situation	Tube restraint target-biting	Unfamiliar	Test animal	20	i.p.	0.5	—
									1.0, 2.0	↓

Notes: Apart from tube-testing situations, all models are of paired interactions. All test animals were male, except where indicated (*) where females were employed, and (+) where both males and females were used. **Dixon, private communication.
Key as for Table 4.1.

other activities (e.g. rearing and approaching) unchanged.[73] Interestingly, if alcohol is given to the group-housed opponent rather than the isolated resident, the same behavioural changes are seen in the non-drugged isolates. These changes are most pronounced when both animals are simultaneously treated with alcohol.[73] Similar findings in other studies on mice have been reported,[74] but recently it has been claimed that untreated resident mice show increased aggression towards alcohol-treated intruders.[75,76] Both studies reported dose-dependent increases in attack by untreated residents, although the latter showed a significant effect only at the highest dose (3.0g/kg). This dose did not decrease locomotor activity, but suppressed rearing and upright defensive behaviour, presumably rendering the mice incapable of showing appropriate defensive responses. In the same study, resident rats increased their attack on intruders treated with 1.7g/kg, but lower doses were ineffective. These workers claim their findings are relevant to the human situation, where high levels of aggression may be directed towards individuals whose behaviour is altered by alcohol[76] (see also Evans and Coid, this volume).

'Interactional' effects in which one member of a pair of male rats is separated from its partner for 24 hours and then re-introduced into the home cage promoting social activity, have been examined.[77,78,79] The removed animal was given moderate to high doses of alcohol 30 min before its re-introduction. Aggression and most other social acts were decreased in treated rats, and 'defence' was reduced by the highest dose. The decreased aggression may not be a specific action since all upright or bipedal postures (including 'full aggressive posture'[80]) were suppressed; alcohol may simply render the animal unable to raise the upper part of the body, rather than change its emotionality. Untreated rats showed fewer defensive postures and full aggressive postures in response to alcohol-treated partners. These changes may, in turn, produce indirect changes in the behaviour of the alcohol-treated partner. For example, the decrease in aggressive postures in untreated rats may cause the decreased frequency of defensive postures in intoxicated animals. This demonstrates the complexity of effects of alcohol in social situations, where the behaviour of the treated animal may be directly (pharmacologically) affected by the drug, and the altered response of the untreated partner may further change the recipient's behaviour.

A much lower dose of alcohol than was used in previous studies

(0.5g/kg) was found to *increase* the frequency and duration of aggressive activities in male isolated mice paired for 10 minutes with untreated (Dixon, private communication), isolated conspecifics.[81] Alcohol also increased flight behaviour, although no distinction was made between passive and active flight[82] (passive flight describes the defensive acts and postures which are made in response to an aggressive partner, whilst active flight occurs when interacting with non-aggressive partners[83]). These low-dose aggression-elevating effects of alcohol were confirmed using individually housed male mice tested in encounters with non-aggressive group-housed opponents.[82] Untreated isolates were initially rated as 'aggressive', 'sociable' or 'timid' in encounters with group-housed intruders. A biphasic effect on aggression in 'aggressive' isolates in subsequent drug trials was evident, with the frequency of 'aggressive unrests' increased at the lowest dose (0.4g/kg) and suppressed by higher doses (0.8 to 2.4g/kg). This demonstrates again the narrow range of low doses that seemingly increase aggression. 'Attack' was not actually potentiated at any dose, but was suppressed at higher doses. Ethanol had no effect on aggression in 'sociable' isolates, but 'timid' mice showed increases in all measures of aggression at 0.8g/kg; these activities were unaffected at lower and higher doses (although suppressions would not easily be observed, since the initial baselines were very low). Alcohol generally failed to reduce timidity and was categorised as a relatively potent aggression-stimulating drug in male mice, although only in mice which showed agonistic behaviour (i.e. aggression or timid/defensive responses) in non-drug screening trials. The behavioural effects observed after drug administration are thus highly dependent upon the nature of the recipient; indeed, the same dose (0.8g/kg) may potentiate aggression in some subjects (timid mice), but reduce it in others (aggressive mice). Not all aspects of aggression were potentiated at a given dose of alcohol in all situations; e.g. 'aggressive unrest' was the only element increased in 'aggressive' mice. Doubt has been cast whether 'aggressive unrest' (walking around the partner, chasing it or walking on its own axis) really is a good index of aggressive tendencies.[24] A factor analysis of murine agonistic behaviour revealed that activity directed toward the partner did not correlate with more traditional measures of aggression, such as biting and tail-rattling.[84]

The effects of alcohol on aggression have been examined in

isolated male rats, trained to traverse a tunnel for a food reward.[85] After four to six weeks of training, aggressive behaviour was measured by placing rats at opposite ends of the tunnel, allowing one rat to force the other back into its starting box and then closing the tunnel. Fighting usually occurred in the absence of food reinforcement. Dominant rats were given low or moderate doses of alcohol 10 min before a 15-min test against a non-drugged subordinate animal. Attack frequency and aggressive posture duration both increased at the low dose (0.5g/kg), although not all aggressive activities were potentiated ('allogrooming' or 'aggressive' grooming showed no such increase). The higher dose (1.0g/kg) non-significantly 'suppressed' attack, and defence was unchanged. Subordinate rats were similarly tested by pairing such animals with non-drugged dominant opponents.[85] They showed no potentiation or suppression of aggression at any dose (the lack of suppression was likely to be due to the low baselines). Alcohol-treated subordinates were threatened more frequently by their non-drugged partners, but the latency to attack them increased. Tests using naîve (rather than subordinate) animals treated with alcohol resulted in their being attacked and injured more frequently than controls, but there was no potentiation of their own aggressive behaviour. Aggression was thus only potentiated in previously aggressive animals; the facilitation of ongoing aggression may not, however, indicate an extraordinary aggression-stimulating potency.[82] It is perhaps less likely that increases in aggression of previously non-aggressive animals would be observed in this study,[85] since these animals were tested against dominant rats (cf previous studies using non-aggressive opponents throughout[82]).

The effect of alcohol on 'suppressed' social conflict aggression in mice has also been examined.[86] Reproductively experienced male mice were paired against a group-housed opponent, either in the resident's home cage or a neutral cage. Under control treatments, attack frequencies were approximately 50 per cent lower in neutral cages than in home cages (hence the 'suppressed' aggression). Mice treated with low to moderate doses of alcohol acutely, and tested in their home cages, had unchanged aggressive and defensive behaviours. In tests conducted in neutral cages, however, alcohol increased attack and sideways threat (but not tail-rattle) at a low dose (0.3g/kg), and decreased sideways threat at a higher dose (1.2g/kg), illustrating a biphasic effect on one aspect (sideways threat) of suppressed aggression. The results suggest that alcohol increases aggression by disinhibiting subjects from showing such responses, but does not directly stimulate aggressive behaviour. As attack increased at a low dose with no change in non-agonistic postures, the results do not support a general activation or increase in arousal.[86] The postulated specific effect on suppressed aggression, might however, simply be a consequence of the rate-dependency of alcohol's effects on aggression, i.e. it may elevate low rates of aggression but leave higher rates unaffected.

These results lead one to examine methodologies employed in rodent studies that have claimed potentiations of aggression by alcohol: many were *not* carried out in the home cage[61,82,85] and may also involve 'suppressed' aggression. Recently, however, it has been claimed that ethanol doses of 0.5 and 1.0g/kg increase attack and sideways threat posture in mice tested with non-drugged group-housed intruders in the *home* cage of the resident,[75] a finding in marked contrast to the previous study.[86] A dose of 2.0g/kg suppressed attack in this situation. Nevertheless, 'suppressed' aggression seems an important feature of alcohol/aggression studies, and recent work has investigated other models of this behaviour.[87,88] In one such study,[88] ethanol's effects were examined on individually housed male mice in dyadic encounters with female intruders, a situation which produces marked suppression of aggression in mice.[89] Obviously, sexual motivation is likely to predominate in such encounters, but an active suppression of social aggression shown towards female mice by males may be related to an olfactory inhibition of aggression by female urine.[90] Videotape analysis of encounters revealed that there was *no* potentiation of aggression at any dose tested (0.5 to 2.0g/kg) and the highest dose produced a decrease in this activity. This lack of an aggression-potentiating effect by low alcohol doses has also been reported in further models of 'suppressed' aggression, e.g. maternal attack on male intruders in the absence of the litter, and in isolated males tested in neutral arenas.[72,87] Low doses of alcohol do not invariably lead to increases in 'suppressed' aggression.

Although most rodent studies have used relatively short periods of behavioural observation, some experiments have concerned the long-term or 'delayed' effects of single doses of alcohol on aggression.[91] Male mice were placed individually either side of a partitioned cage for three days prior to testing. Fifteen minutes after alcohol administration the partition was removed, and the squeaks emitted by the mice were automatically recorded by squeal-detection circuits[92] for a period of 23 hours; such squeals have been correlated with fighting frequency and the time spent fighting.[93] One hour after commencement, alcohol at low and moderate doses given to both interacting mice suppressed aggression; the effect remained significant for the moderate dose group 13 hours after the start. Without simultaneous measurements of other aspects of behaviour, it is difficult to distinguish a selective drug effect on aggression from non-specific sedation, although it is unlikely that doses as low as 0.4g/kg are sedative.[94] The findings seem compatible with long-term effects of acute alcohol on target-biting in rats.[69]

Behavioural specificity of the anti-aggressive effect is an important issue in studies relating alcohol to aggressive behaviour.[85] Some previous studies record that many 'anti-aggressive' effects of alcohol are attributable to motor dysfunctions,[77] and it is sometimes claimed that a specific aggression-decreasing effect is unlikely as the doses that reduce aggression are close to those that produce general sedation and ataxia.[83] Selective decreases in aggression may follow moderately high alcohol doses,[73] but recently well-defined specific suppressions of fighting have been shown to occur at very low doses in mice.[95] Naîve, individually housed males treated with alcohol 20 min before a 500-s encounter in their home cage with a non-drugged 'standard opponent'[96,97] showed extended latencies to attack the intruder and decreased durations and frequencies of most aggressive acts and postures with increasing ethanol dose. Some activities (sideways offensive and attack) were depressed even by the lowest alcohol dose (0.1g/kg). The suppression of aggression was not due to a non-specific depression since some bipedal postures (requiring effective motor coordination) were greatly potentiated even at the highest dose (1.0g/kg). Timid/defensive (active flight) activities were increased by alcohol administration at all doses. This is in marked contrast to claims that defensive and flight behaviour are largely unaffected by alcohol at non-ataxic doses.[82,86]

Alcohol at low, moderate and high doses selectively suppressed aggression in 'aggressively-rated' individually housed Swiss and TO strain mice tested 20 min after drug application with a non-drugged 'standard opponent'.[98,99] Swiss mice were more sensitive to alcohol, showing decreases in aggression and increases in timid/

defensive behaviour at lower doses, i.e. the effective doses may be quite different in different strains of mice. The high baselines of fighting would not facilitate observation of potentiations of aggression (even though increases in such activities have been reported in aggressive animals[82,85]), but even the supposedly 'aggression-potentiating' dose of 0.5g/kg produced a clear anti-aggressive effect in this situation. As already noted, an aggression-stimulating dose in some subjects may suppress these same activities in other animals.[82]

Attempts have been made[24,25] to determine whether alcohol potentiates aggression via a disinhibition (i.e. removal of a learned inhibition against aggressive responding) or via a 'direct' stimulation of fighting behaviour. Individually housed male TA (Turku Aggressive) and TNA (Turku Non-aggressive) strain mice were used. Each TA mouse was trained to non-aggression by being repeatedly defeated by a highly aggressive opponent, whilst the genetically non-aggressive TNA mice needed no such training. It was argued that if alcohol potentiates aggression via disinhibition, only the alcohol-treated TA mice (having a learned inhibition of aggression) would show increases, whilst if the drug acted via direct stimulation, both TA and TNA would show enhanced levels of fighting. Mice were given a moderately high dose of ethanol 15 min before a 7-min trial against a 'standard opponent'[100] in the isolate's home cage. There were no differences between alcohol- and saline-treated groups in either TA or TNA mice. Repeating the experiment using more animals, a more severe training of TA animals to non-aggression, and applying two moderately high doses of alcohol (1.0 and 1.5g/kg), produced no increase in aggression.

It was suggested[24] that these results support neither the disinhibition nor the direct stimulation hypotheses. Indeed, it was argued that 'animals cannot be used as models to explain the increased violence in humans under the influence of alcohol intoxication'. The doses used were somewhat higher than those usually reported to potentiate aggression (they are usually lower than 0.8g/kg), and fall into the dose range that has frequently been shown to suppress aggression. The doses were not however inordinately high (they were considered high enough to have an effect, but not to impair motor activity[101]), underlining the point that low doses of ethanol that are reported to potentiate aggression are *very* low and cover a very narrow range. The (presumed) aggression-elevating effects in humans seemingly occur over an extremely wide range of alcohol levels.[23] Some idea of how low the aggression-stimulating doses in animals are, may be illustrated by considering the BAC after acute administration of such doses. For example, the BAC measured 20 min after an intraperitoneal injection of 0.5g/kg of alcohol in Swiss mice was just 25mg/100ml.[98] Even allowing for differential sensitivity to similar BACs, it is evident that such concentrations are very low in human terms (80mg/100ml is the current British legal driving limit). The effectiveness of such low doses may, however, be a consequence of the relative naïvety of test animals to alcohol exposure. Humans are generally more experienced in this respect.

Studies on acute alcohol administration in rodents use a range of strains and species, a variety of routes of alcohol administration (together with varying times after administration), different testing conditions (e.g. testing in the light[86] or the dark parts[98] of the light/dark cycle), employ home or neutral arenas, different types of opponent, and utilise a wide range of behavioural models of aggression. Even within studies using the same means of eliciting 'aggression', methodologies can be highly variable, e.g. in the 'isolation-induced' paradigm, periods of individual housing vary from several days[91] up to ten months.[25] Both duration of isolation and the age at which isolation commences markedly influence subsequent fighting behaviour in mice,[102] making comparisons between studies difficult. It is perhaps not too surprising to note apparently divergent results on 'aggression', since the effect observed under the influence of alcohol is likely to depend on a combination of factors. Certain variables seem of particular importance, e.g. the type of testing arena employed seems important, as most studies reporting increases in aggression tested the animals in neutral or unfamiliar arenas,[61,82,85,86] whilst those reporting decreases or no effect at similar doses, generally used home cages.[24,25,91,95,98] Perhaps alcohol is more likely to potentiate aggression when it has been experimentally suppressed (thus disinhibiting the subject) rather than directly stimulating aggression? This is not the only important variable, however, as a number of studies on various forms of suppressed aggression have revealed no potentiation of these activities by alcohol.[72,87,88]

The behavioural baseline of the activity being studied at the time a drug becomes active often determines the effect of treatment.[103,104] This may be a factor in some rodent studies which have shown alcohol to suppress fighting in animals with high baselines, whilst the same low doses potentiate this activity in animals with lower baselines.[82] On the other hand, animals with both high *and* low baselines have been reported to show low-dose potentiations or lack of potentiation.[82,87,98]

Reports failing to show potentiation of aggression by alcohol generally use 'standard opponents',[24,25,87,95,98] whereas potentiations are often recorded when 'non-aggressive' group-housed animals or (presumably aggressive) isolates are used. 'Standard opponents' are docile, never initiating fighting nor showing signs of overt aggression; fighting is consequently unidirectional, and thus more accurately reflects the experimental manipulation of the test animal.[105,106] Differential effects of alcohol on aggression may partially result from using different types of opponent. Indeed, extrapolating between tests using different types of intruder may be inappropriate, the use of different types of 'standard opponent' can produce significant changes in the behaviour of non-drugged resident mice.[105]

Studies employing relatively long interludes between acute drug administration and testing consistently record suppressions of aggression, even at low doses.[69,91] No studies on potential long-term increases in aggressive behaviour after acute alcohol administration have been located. The aggression-elevating effect if it occurs, thus appears to be a relatively short-duration phenomenon.

Most rodent studies include no blood-alcohol data, making extrapolations difficult. Animals tested 10 min after alcohol administration are likely to have very different BACs from animals tested after 30 min, even if the same dose is used. This is particularly true of lower ethanol doses. Indeed, mice injected i.p. with 0.5g/kg show zero BACs 60 min after application (Figure 4.1). Simple experimental manipulations such as varying the housing condition (e.g. isolated v. group-housed) can result in different BACs after the same dose of alcohol.[107] Animals of varying weight and size produce markedly different BACs even after i.p. injections of the *same* alcohol dose.[108] Different routes of alcohol administration may also produce different BACs at similar times after administration (Figure 4.2): the rate of distribution to the site of action of a drug tends to be slower when administered p.o. rather than i.p.[109] The route of administration *per se* does not appear to explain confounding results on aggression, however, as increases, decreases or lack of effect on this attribute have been

Figure 4.1: Mean Blood-Alcohol Levels Measured at Various Times After Acute i.p. Injections of Three Doses of Alcohol in Male, Swiss-strain Mice (▲ = 0.5, ● = 1.0 and ■ = 2.0g/kg body wt)

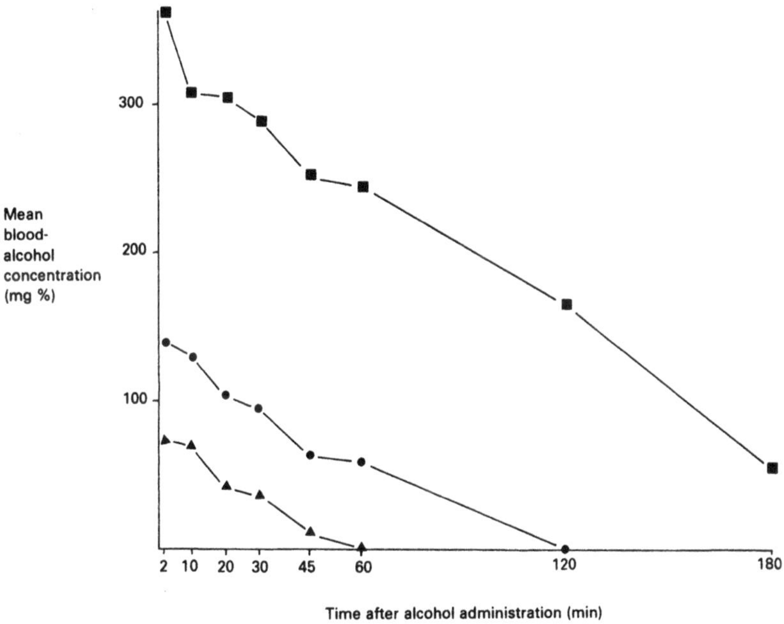

reported with comparable alcohol doses using either the i.p. or p.o. application. Clearly, measurement of BACs at the time of testing would facilitate more meaningful comparisons between different studies on alcohol and infra-human aggression.

The data for these studies are summarised in Table 4.5.

(3) *Self-administration of Alcohol in Rodents*

Relatively few studies examine giving alcohol to rodents as a dilute solution in the drinking water and then assessing aggression. Such self-administration has been used in studies on territorial behaviour of male mice.[110] Territories ($1.8m^2$) were partitioned into halves, and four mice placed on each side. After one week the partition was removed, and it was noted which mouse eventually became despot over the whole enclosure. When a 5 per cent alcohol solution was provided for the mice on one side of the partition for three days prior to the removal, the dominant mouse of the

Figure 4.2: Mean Blood-Alcohol Levels Measured 20 Min After i.p. or p.o. Administration of 0.5g/kg Ethanol in Swiss Mice

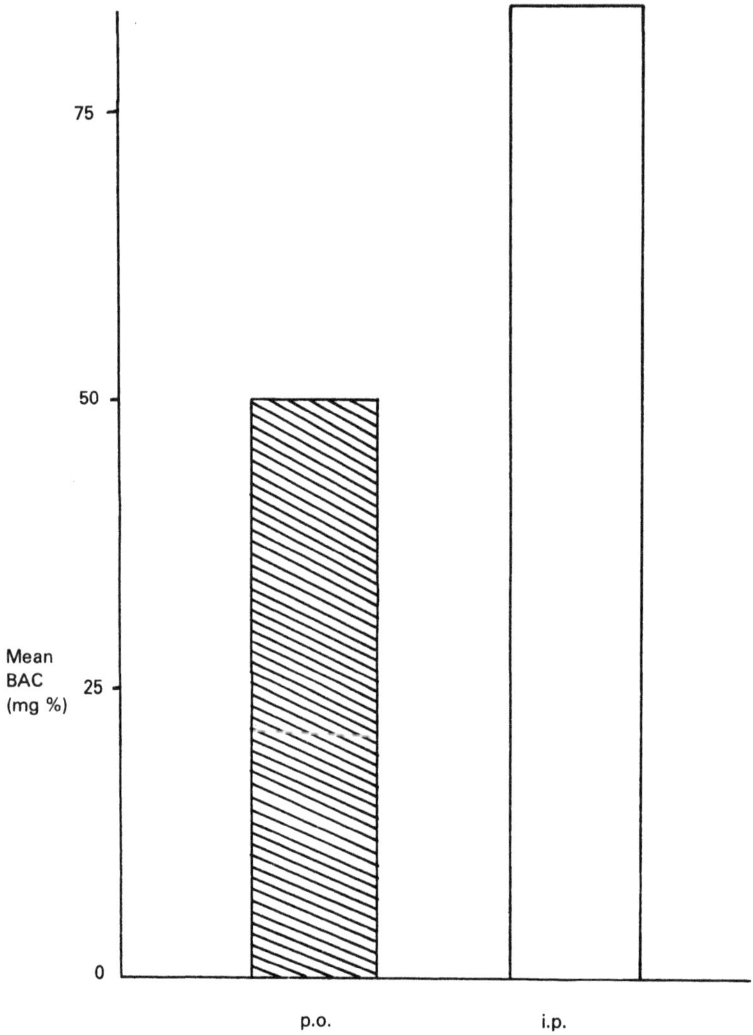

alcohol-treated group eventually became despot over the whole enclosure (usually within three to five days). No effect was evident if alcohol was given one week after the partition was removed.

Effects of alcohol administered in the drinking water have also been studied on social interactions of group-housed mice in encounters with non-drugged females.[110] One group of males received 10 per cent alcohol for three days prior to testing, whilst controls received water. An unfamiliar male and female were placed together in a neutral arena. There were no effects on aggression or flight, but social and sexual activities increased, suggesting that alcohol generally potentiates the type of behaviour which is stimulated by the test situation.

The effects of long-term administration of alcohol and its subsequent withdrawal have also been studied.[111] Male group-housed mice were given water or 8 per cent alcohol to drink for seven days before testing. Mice were paired (treated v. non-treated) in a neutral arena and social interactions observed for 5 min. Aggression and flight were unchanged in alcohol-exposed subjects compared to untreated partners. Alcohol administration was continued for a total of 21 days (the average daily intake was approximately 12g/kg over this time), and then replaced by water. Twenty-four hours later, mice were paired as before, and aggression was seen to be unchanged, whereas flight was increased (mainly due to an increase in 'flagging'). Withdrawal reactions were generally fairly mild compared to reactions in other studies.[112]

These few studies using alcohol administration via the drinking water provide little support for this drug having a potent aggression-stimulating effect. Only the greater probability of an alcohol-treated dominant male eventually becoming the despot in the territorial dominance situation supports this view. As the experiment was repeated only four times, the fact that the alcohol-treated dominant became the despot on all occasions is not very impressive.

Data for these studies are summarised in Table 4.6.

Alcohol and Aggression in Cats

Studies on cats have frequently examined 'aggressive' behaviour elicited by electrical stimulation of the brain. The effects of alcohol on 'sham rage', elicited by stimulation of the hypothalamus[113] have been studied. This behaviour is characterised by pupil dilation, claw extrusion, piloerection, baring of the teeth, lashing of the tail and fighting. Low concentrations of intracerebrally administered

Table 4.6: Effect of Alcohol Given in the Drinking Water on Aggression in Rodents

Authors	Animal	Age	Behavioural test	Arena	Alcohol concentration in drinking water	Time of test after start of alcohol treatment (days)	Drug recipient	Effect on aggression
110	CFW mice		Group interaction: alcohol-treated v. non-alcohol treated group	Home	5%	3 days prior to 'pairing' groups	1 group	(↑)
						7 days after 'pairing' groups	1 group	—
		10-12 weeks	Paired interaction: male v. group-housed female	Unfamiliar	10%	3	Test animal	—
		12 weeks	Paired interaction: male v. group-housed male	Unfamiliar	5%	10	Both animals	(↓)
111	CFLP mice	18 weeks	Paired interaction: male v. group-housed male	Unfamiliar	8%	7	Test animal	—
						21 days, then 1 day's withdrawal	Test animal	—

Notes: All subjects were group-housed males. Alcohol was given in the drinking water.
Key as for Table 4.1.

alcohol slightly stimulated such behaviour (as evidenced by a lowered response threshold to electrical stimulation), whilst higher doses suppressed. Intravenous administration of alcohol depressed the electrically stimulated motor responses of the cortex. The emotional mimetic reactions of the hypothalamus were unchanged or increased in both intensity and duration. The project was terminated, however, as it was thought to lack behavioural significance:[114] e.g. sham rage can occur in decerebrate cats in which the entire forebrain is removed.[115]

Recent studies have examined alcohol's effects on more easily controlled forms of aggression that can be induced by brain stimulation. A pattern of precisely coordinated predatory behaviour involving minimal sympathetic display and described as 'quiet biting attack'[116,117] has been used.[118] The duration and intensity of this behaviour is easily controlled by varying the neural stimulation. Attacks were elicited by stimulating the hypothalamus using chronically implanted electrodes, with the resulting 'aggression' being directed towards an anaesthetised rat. After a number of control trials in which the cat was stimulated to make quiet biting predatory attacks, alcohol was administered directly into the blood via a jugular catheter. This produced a dose-dependent increase in attack latency, affecting all four behavioural phases (initial arousal, movement towards prey object, orientation of head to target and finally seizure of the prey object). The major effects involved the last three phases, particularly seizure of the prey object, which may be partially accounted for by reduced motor output of the mechanisms controlling jaw activity.[119] Difficulties in jaw opening and head orientation were noted, together with delayed approaches to the target. The force of biting increased, however, particularly at the higher alcohol doses — an increase in force of jaw closure became apparent even at low doses of 0.25g/kg. Thus, there were aspects of both potentiation and attenuation of predatory attack, and the results suggested that brain-stimulated aggression was a good model for studying the neural bases of alcohol's modulation of 'aggressive' behaviour.

The effects of alcohol on 'affective defence'[120,121] have also been studied in cats.[122] Here, the animal assumes threatening postures and attacks a conspecific with its claws in a highly coordinated fashion. Although there is much sympathetic display, including hissing, spitting, and raising of the hackles, affective defence is unlike sham rage in that the animal is more responsive to its environment. These responses were obtained by electrical stimulation of the hypothalamic ventromedial nucleus (VM), using chronically implanted electrodes. Cats were restrained in head-holders and subjected to electrical stimulation of the VM, producing hissing responses (even in the absence of an appropriate 'target' animal, although such responses have a shorter latency in the presence of a conspecific). Hissing latency was considered as an index of VM excitation. A 'target' cat was placed in front of the restrained subject and the electrical stimulus strength adjusted until a hissing latency of between 7 and 10 seconds was obtained. A biphasic response to ethanol was obtained, with low doses reducing and higher doses increasing this measure. Although it is a possibility, the authors suggest that one would not be justified to conclude that low doses of alcohol arouse hostile behaviour in cats in normal (unstimulated) encounters with conspecifics, as such activities are influenced by many neural factors.

The effects of alcohol on defensive behaviour have also been examined in a free-interaction situation.[123,124] Defensive behaviour included several 'aggressive' components such as hissing, fighting and biting, and was elicited by presenting the alcohol-treated subject with a 'stimulus' cat in a neutral arena. The 'stimulus' cat was neurally stimulated via electrodes implanted in the hypothalamus, producing various degrees of aggressive response, including alerting, threat and attack. The subject's responses to these activities were recorded on a rating scale. A biphasic response to ethanol was also evident here. Low doses of alcohol (0.25g/kg) enhanced overall defensive behaviour, but no individual component of the behavioural repertoire was potentiated. Slightly higher doses (0.5 to 1.0g/kg) left aggressive behaviour unchanged, and 1.5g/kg depressed such activities.

Work on cats generally reveals excitatory effects of alcohol at low doses, with depressant effects at higher doses. The work appears unique among studies on alcohol and infra-human aggression in employing direct electrical brain-stimulation techniques.

Data for these studies are summarised in Table 4.7.

Alcohol and Aggression in Dogs

Dogs seem useful experimental animals in alcohol research since

Table 4.7: Effect of Alcohol on Aggression in Cats

Authors	Animal	Age	Sex	Behavioural test	Arena	Time after admini-stration	Route of admini-stration	Ethanol dose	Effect on aggression
113	Cat			Electrically stimulated 'sham rage'			i.c.	~ 0.016mg	(↑)
								~ 0.032mg	—
								~ 0.047 to 0.789mg	↓
							i.v.	0.79-2.37g/kg	↑
118	Cat			Electrically stimulated 'quiet biting' predatory attack on rat	Unfamiliar	10	i.v.	0.37, 0.75, 1.5g/kg	↑↓
122	Cat	Adult	Female	Electrically stimulated 'affective defence' in presence of conspecific	Unfamiliar	0	i.v.	0.37g/kg	↑
								1.5g/kg	↓
123	Cat		Male	Paired interaction-test animal v. male conspecific electrically stimulated to aggression	Unfamiliar	20	i.p.	0.25g/kg	↑
								0.5, 1.0g/kg	—
								1.5g/kg	↓

Note: Key as for Table 4.1.

litters form social hierarchies[125,126] which tend to be stable and difficult to disrupt experimentally.[127] Aggressive, dominant individuals occupy high ranks in those social orders, whilst the bottom ranks are timid, inhibited, dominated animals. Between these extremes are dogs which dominate submissive animals, but are dominated by the most aggressive animals.[128] Food intake in a competitive situation has been studied in a hierarchy of four Dalmation–Setter F_1 hybrids, the group consisting of one female and three male animals.[128] When only one animal was able to feed at any one time (from a food pan covered by a wooden box with a single head-hole in it), the subordinate animal obtained very restricted quantities of food. Conflict often arose between dominant animals in food competition tests, but generally the 'frustrations' engendered were displaced to the subordinate, which was frequently bitten and attacked even when it was remote from the food source. It has been suggested that this indicates an emotional outlet following conflict and frustration.[128] The subordinate animal developed a conditioned fear reaction which inhibited its responses in the presence of attackers. It was argued that if these inhibiting factors could be removed by a drug, the submissive animal might show more aggression, resulting in increased food intake in the competitive situation. Giving the subordinate dog a low dose of alcohol (0.43g/kg), 8 to 10 min before competitive feeding experiments, resulted in its becoming more aggressive. The time spent in the immediate vicinity of the pan and the amount of food consumed were also both increased. Alcohol may have stimulated appetite (any dogs given alcohol show increased food intake) rather than aggression *per se*, but 'aggressive' behaviour was not seen on other days when the animal seemed ravenously hungry. It was concluded that alcohol removes cerebral inhibition, generating more aggressive behaviour, and such processes may account for increases in aggression in humans as well as dogs.

Ethanol's effects have also been assessed on social behaviour in groups of three Telomian dogs, each group consisting of two males and one female.[129] These were considered good subjects for aggression studies as they show high frequencies of agonistic threats.[130] Canine dominance tests[131] were given in which pairs of dogs were given a bone, and the individual controlling it for the longer period was considered dominant. The present experiment used an artificial rawhide 'bone' as a standard stimulus for eliciting agonistic behaviour. Alcohol was given to no one or all dogs in the group at a given dose. The low dose (0.8g/kg) increased attack frequency and bone-possession time in the lowest ranked dogs, whilst highest and intermediate ranked individuals actually showed decreases in these measures when given the same dose of ethanol. Higher doses of alcohol decreased all these measures in all individuals. Similar findings occurred whether one or all of the interacting animals received alcohol. Both doses of alcohol decreased agonistic vocalisation frequency. Alcohol was thus able to temporarily disrupt a dominance hierarchy, which has been noted to be remarkably stable.[127] It had different effects on different members of the social group; potentiation of aggression principally occurred in submissive animals in both canine studies.

Data for these studies on dogs are summarised in Table 4.8.

Alcohol and Aggression in Monkeys

Studies on primates have concentrated on the effects of alcohol on Rhesus and Pigtail macaques (*Macaca spp.*). Monkeys are potentially useful subjects as they form hierarchical social structures which are fairly stable.[132,133] The most dominant monkey tends to set the overall pattern of the hierarchy, with different monkeys following its lead and responding deferentially according to their position in the structure.[134] It has been suggested that the Rhesus monkey is a particularly appropriate model since its physiology,[135] social organisation and behaviour bear a resemblance to those of man.[136]

Individual and social behaviour both before and after voluntary consumption of alcohol were studied in a colony of four adult male Rhesus monkeys[137] (*Macaca mulatta*). Animals were observed in a large colony cage for 14 days prior to alcohol administration, and the social hierarchy determined. There was one overall dominant who established his position by activities such as pushing, pulling and biting the other animals, one clear subordinate (to all colony members) and two individuals of intermediate status. After the last day of social observations, animals were individually housed for nine days and allowed to drink in a free choice situation either alcohol diluted in a cherry-flavoured drink, or the flavoured drink alone. The lowest-ranked monkey drank most alcohol and was the most active and aggressive — it forcibly pushed out four drinking

Table 4.8: Effect of Alcohol on Aggression in Dogs

Authors	Animal	Age	Sex	Type	Behavioural test	Drug recipient	Time after administration (min)	Ethanol dose (g/kg)	Effect on aggression
128	Dalmatian-Setter F_1 hybrids	< 85 days	Male and female	Male Gp subordinate	Group competitive feeding situation	Test animal	8-10	0.43	↑
129	Telomian dogs	< 67 days	Male and female	Gp subordinate	Group competitive bone-possession situation	Test animal or all animals	40-80	0.8 1.6	↑ (↓) ↓
				Gp dominant	Group competitive bone-possession situation	Test animal or all animals	40-80	0.8 1.6	↓

Note: In each case alcohol was administered directly into the stomach, and tests took place in an unfamiliar arena.
Key as for Table 4.1.

bottles and broke them, which was taken to be consistent with increased aggressivity (!). When the monkeys were returned to their colony cage, although the previous dominant retained his position, the formerly lowest-ranked individual was now second in the social hierarchy, and became much more aggressive and socially active. Alcohol consumption remained high in the now 2nd-ranked monkey, perhaps indicating the importance of the drug in helping him maintain his new-found status. Alcohol consumption dropped in the now 3rd and 4th-ranked monkeys, but subsequently increased in one individual. Alcohol consumption can markedly influence the social roles and relationships in Rhesus monkeys, and the findings illustrate individual differences in the response to alcohol, which also seem characteristic of humans.

Alcohol's effects have been studied in a colony of four adolescent male Rhesus monkeys, to determine whether enough alcohol would be consumed voluntarily in a social situation to induce intoxication, and to observe the subsequent effects on social behaviour.[136] Monkeys were housed in a large colony cage and social contact activities (mounting, huddling, grooming and playing, including mauling, biting and wrestling) were observed in 20-min sessions. Once a dominance hierarchy had been established, observations of normal social behaviour were made for 21 days. Subsequently, monkeys were provided with orange juice, and a mixture of ethanol and orange juice for 40 min, which corresponded to the first 40 min of an 80-min observation period. One hour later, a further 20-min period of observation was made. Alcohol concentration in the orange juice was 2 per cent v/v for three consecutive days, but increased to 3, then 4, 5, 6 and eventually 7 per cent v/v for blocks of three consecutive days at each concentration. Solutions were voluntarily consumed and, although the volume of fluid intake decreased as a function of the alcohol concentration, the net intake of alcohol tended to remain stable. Alcohol increased play and walking along a metal bar (although more failures in crossings were noted, indicating (a) ataxia and (b) that monkeys would voluntarily consume sufficient alcohol to become intoxicated). The increase in play activity may be due to an overall increase in activity (as suggested by increased bar crossings). As bar crossings occur in play behaviour and there were no significant differences on other measures, the data are inconclusive. It was suggested that the social structure of the group changed as a result of alcohol intake, as increased play activity tends to be associated with a deterioration of the dominance hierarchy.[138] When dominant animals become intoxicated the hierarchy may deteriorate, relaxing social restraints and facilitating social interactions. The study did not find increases in aggression or timidity.

The effects of alcohol have been studied on five adult male Pigtail macaques (*M. nemestrina*) belonging to a troop of about 30 individuals.[139] All studied subjects ranked immediately below the dominant male, and low to moderate ethanol doses were given by nasogastric intubation (a tube from the nose to the stomach). After alcohol administration, animals were returned to the colony, and observed 15 min later for a total period of 55 min during the following three hours. Frequencies of nine dominance (including threat, pursuit and biting[140]) and nine submissive (such as grimacing, withdrawal and flight) activities were recorded. Alcohol had no measurable effect on submission or dominance but increased 'playful fighting' at higher doses, a behaviour usually typical of juveniles. Such fighting is unlike true fighting in that although prolonged wrestling may occur, animals are uninjured, and withdrawal, flight and submission are not seen. These results seem compatible with the increases in play observed in other primate studies.[136] It is highly questionable whether increases in playful fighting are analogous to the types of violence said to be augmented in humans under the influence of alcohol. The authors suggested that since violence does not follow alcohol intake in some cultures, the drug's influence on aggression may be more cultural than pharmacological. They suggest that data from this animal model lend experimental support to anthropological studies[141] indicating that there is little direct pharmacological effect of ethanol on human aggression.

Studies on social behaviour of primates do not support the view that alcohol has marked aggression-elevating effect. Aggression was increased in one individual in one study,[137] but may have been an indirect effect of alcohol's action on the formerly intermediate-ranked animals who declined in rank. Alcohol influences, however, both individual and social behaviour in primates, to the extent that even the dominance hierarchy and social structure may be altered. Only earlier studies where (a) chronic alcohol administration was used, and (b) all animals received the drug simultaneously, showed such effects.[136,137] Changes in social hierarchies have not been observed in studies where alcohol is administered to a single member of the colony. It is also possible that drug effects on social behaviour may depend on the stability of the investigated social groups.[139]

The effects of alcohol have been studied on 'self-aggression',[142] an abnormal behaviour which is said to develop as a result of 'frustration'.[143] Adult males which are individually housed show such responses. Four individually housed, mature Rhesus macaques with strong self-aggressive tendencies acted as experimental subjects, whilst similar monkeys acted as controls. Alcohol (5 to 15 per cent v/v) in orange juice was consumed voluntarily over a two-month testing period. Animals were tested after *ad libitum* intake of alcohol, or after a period of fluid deprivation followed by rapid intake of alcohol (in order to increase the alcohol intake just prior to testing). The latency, frequency and duration of self-biting and self-slapping behaviour were recorded in response to threatening gestures performed by the experimenter,[144] including hitting the front of the cage and 'pulling threatening faces'. Latency and frequency of the animals' responses were unaltered, but there was a dose-dependent increase in the duration of self-aggression after alcohol administration.

Further studies have examined the emotional responses of primates to the experimenter.[145] Three individuals of one sub-species of *M. nemestrina* were compared directly to two individuals of another sub-species, all animals receiving the same treatment. Subjects were individually housed for seven days of adaptation in cages supplied with two drinking bottles. The water supply was then replaced by an alcohol solution for four days and, finally one bottle was replaced with water giving the animals a free choice (alcohol or water). Alcohol selection was monitored for 15 weeks, and there were marked differences in the preferences of the two sub-species. Alcohol solutions were replaced by water for the 16th and 17th weeks, and measures of emotionality made during the 15th and 17th weeks. Aggressive and non-aggressive activities displayed in response to the investigator[146] were determined at 2-s intervals, for 120 s per day for each subject. The sub-species that showed the greater alcohol preference exhibited less fearful behaviour and more aggression. After withdrawal of the alcohol solution, these animals showed a 50 per cent reduction in aggressive behaviour, but levels were still elevated compared to the other sub-species. There were consequently differences in emotional behaviour which correlated with ethanol selection. NB there was no indication that the two sub-species showed pre-treatment differences in 'emotionality'.

The effects of cortical ablations were assessed on ethanol selection and emotionality in female Pigtail macaques.[147] Prior to the study, subjects received bilateral dorsolateral or orbital frontal lesions of the cortex, surgery known to affect 'emotional' responses.[146,148] Alcohol selection of subjects was measured daily as the amount of ethanol solution drunk in a two-bottle choice paradigm. Emotionality was measured by direct observation of aggressive and aversive reactions to the observer. During a total of 8 observations, subjects were 'loaded' with 15ml of 95 per cent ethanol in orange juice on 4 occasions, and 4 times given orange juice only. This was the maximal amount of alcohol animals would voluntarily consume, and produced mild signs of intoxication. Animals with dorsolateral lesions selected ethanol more frequently than did their intact controls, who in turn selected ethanol more frequently than animals with orbital lesions. Dorsolateral ablations increased aggression, an effect potentiated by alcohol. Orbital lesions decreased aggressive behaviour, but alcohol-loading increased such activities. Alcohol tended to increase levels of aggression, and reduce retreats in intact animals. The overall results indicate that alcohol disinhibits emotion and also interacts with the lesion effects.

Studies on 'aggression' in individually housed animals responding to human observers suggest that increased levels of aggressivity are associated with alcohol intake, in contrast to studies on intraspecific social situations. Potentiations are thus only generally seen in long-term isolated monkeys, a condition that cannot be considered as normal for these highly social animals. It has been previously noted, for example, that abnormal activities such as self-aggression are associated with individual housing.[144] The results on more naturalistic situations (which suggest that ethanol can reduce inhibitions of certain activities) may be more representative of the drug's psychopharmacological action on normal social and emotional behaviour.

Data for these studies on primates are summarised in Table 4.9.

Conclusions

In humans, the circumstances of drinking may actually produce

Table 4.9: Effect of Alcohol on Aggression in Monkeys

Authors	Animal	Age	Sex	Type	Behavioural test	Arena	Drug recipient	Time after admini-stration	Route of admini-stration	Ethanol dose	Effect on aggression
137	Rhesus monkey	Mature	Male	Gp, subordinate	Group social interaction	Home	All animals		Orally, free choice	21.7 g/day	↑
				Gp, sub-dominant	Group social interaction	Home	All animals		Orally, free choice	10.5-13.2 g/day	(↓)
				Gp, dominant	Group social interaction	Home	All animals		Orally, free choice	15.9 g/day	—
142	Rhesus monkey	5 years		Is	Self-aggression in response to investigator	Home	Test animal		Orally, voluntarily consumed	Up to 7.9 g/kg/day	↑
136	Rhesus monkey	Adolescent	Male	Gp	Group social interaction	Unfamiliar (but which became home)	All animals	During administration and up to 100 min later	Orally, free choice	~ 16.6 g/day	—
145	Pigtail monkey	4 years		Is, alcohol preferring	Response to investigator	Home	Test animal		Orally, free choice		↑
147	Pigtail monkey	Adult	Female	Is, with brain lesions	Response to investigator	Home	Test animal	30 min	Orally	15ml of 95% ethanol	↑
139	Pigtail monkey	Adult	Male	Gp, sub-dominant	Group social interaction	Home	Test animal	15 min	Nasogastric intubation	0.39-1.6 g/kg	—
76	Squirrel monkey	Adult	Male and female	Gp	Group social interaction	Home	Test animal	5 min	Gavage	0.1, 0.3, 0.6 g/kg	Partners: —
										1.0 g/kg	Partners: —

Key as for Table 4.1.

greater behavioural changes than the intake of alcohol itself.[149] Indeed, the test situation in infra-human animals also tends to markedly affect the observed behaviour under the influence of alcohol. For example, alcohol-induced potentiations of rodent aggression tend generally to occur in neutral rather than home cages. Also, different recipients show differential responses to alcohol. Timid or subordinate animals in social hierarchies tend to show increases in aggression when treated with alcohol. However, doses effective in this respect may actually have an anti-aggressive effect in aggressive or dominant animals. One cannot consequently specify a general aggression-elevating dose even for animals of the same species. Low-dose potentiation of 'aggression' may also occur in fish (although not in a free-interaction situation), cats (where aspects of aggression are elicited by brain stimulation), and neurotic, isolated monkeys responding to an observer. Increases seem mainly to result from disinhibition rather than direct stimulation of aggression. A large number of studies have, however, failed to find a potentiation of aggression by comparable doses of alcohol, suggesting that this substance is *not* a potent aggression-stimulating drug.

Hinde[150] has suggested three possible utilities of animal studies to our understanding of human behaviour. They may:

(1) help one to develop methodologies which can be adapted for use in humans;
(2) be used in particular experiments where ethical considerations preclude the use of humans; and
(3) provide principles or generalisations whose relevance to man can be subsequently assessed.

Studies on the effects of alcohol on aggression that use animal models seems to have all three utilities. It is clear that 'aggression' is a very diverse set of phenomena in both infra-human animals[28] and man.[151] Indeed, it has been suggested[152] that three broad categories of animal aggression, namely: 'social' (competitive, generally ritualised attack including intermale and territorial forms of aggression), 'self-defensive' and 'parental' should be specified. Each of these categories may be influenced differently by biological, situational and experiential factors. It seems inappropriate to extrapolate too freely between different models of attack — a strategy which is certainly unreliable when dealing with the diverse human situations (e.g. homicide, rape, war, refusing to speak etc.) where 'aggression' is said to be involved. Obviously, extrapolating from animals to humans is going to be even more difficult and dangerous. These provisos have been stated, it seems likely that a thorough understanding of the potential association between alcohol administration and behaviour will be facilitated by detailed systematic studies on infra-human animals. Our understanding will be aided by resisting the temptation to over-generalise from any one set of results.

Acknowledgements

R. Smoothy was supported by a Science and Engineering Research Council Studentship.

References

1. Berry, M.S. and Pentreath, V.W. 'The neurophysiology of alcohol' in *Psychopharmacology of Alcohol* (ed Sandler, M.), New York: Raven Press, 1980, pp. 43-72.

2. Lagerspetz, K.M.J. 'Combining aggression studies in infra-humans and man' in *Multidisciplinary Approaches to Aggression Research* (eds Brain, P.F. and Benton, D.), Amsterdam: Elsevier/North-Holland Biomedical Press, 1981, pp. 390-400.

3. Raynes, A.E., Ryback, R. and Ingle, D. 'The effect of alcohol on aggression in *Betta splendens*', *Communications in Behavioral Biology*, 1968, *2*, pp. 141-6.

4. Peeke, H.V.S., Ellman, G.E. and Herz, M.J. 'Dose-dependent alcohol effects on the aggressive behavior of the convict cichlid (*Cichlasoma nigrofasciatum*)', *Behavioral Biology*, 1973, *8*, pp. 115-22.

5. Ryback, R. and Ingle, D. Paper presented at the Eastern Psychological Association Meeting, Washington, DC, 1968.

6. Ryback, R., Percarpio, B. and Vitale, J. 'Equilibration and metabolism of ethanol in the goldfish', *Nature*, 1969, *222*, pp. 1068-70.

7. Raynes, A.E. and Ryback, R.S. 'Effect of alcohol and congeners on aggressive response in *Betta splendens*', *Quarterly Journal of Studies on Alcohol*, 1970, *Suppl. 5*, pp. 130-5.

8. Lissman, H.W. 'Die Umwelt des Kampffiisches (*Betta splendens* Regan)', *Zeitschrift für vergleichende Physiologie*, 1933, *18*, pp. 65-111.

9. Hess, E.H. 'Temperature as a regulator of the attack-response of *Betta splendens*', *Zeitschrift für Tierpsychologie*, 1952, *9*, pp. 379-82.

10. Simpson, M.J.A. 'The display of the Siamese fighting fish, *Betta splendens*', *Animal Behaviour Monographs*, 1968, *1*.

11. Ellman, G.E., Herz, M.J. and Peeke, H.V.S. 'Ethanol in a cichlid fish: blood levels and aggressive behavior', *Proceedings of the Western Pharmacological Society*, 1972, *15*, pp. 92-5.

12. Peeke, H.V.S. and Figler, M.H. 'Modulation of aggressive behavior in fish by alcohol and congeners', *Pharmacology, Biochemistry and Behavior*, 1981, *14, Suppl. 1*, pp. 79-84.

13. Peeke, H.V.S., Peeke, S.C., Avis, H.H. and Ellman, G. 'Alcohol, habituation and the patterning of aggressive responses in a cichlid fish', *Pharmacology, Biochemistry and Behavior*, 1975, *3*, pp. 1031-6.

14. Figler, M.H. and Peeke, H.V.S. 'Alcohol and the prior residence effect in male convict cichlids (*Cichlasoma nigrofasciatum*)', *Aggressive Behavior*, 1978, *4*, pp. 125-32.

15. Braddock, J.C. 'The effect of prior residence upon dominance in the fish *Platypoecilus maculatus*', *Physiological Zoology*, 1949, *22*, pp. 161-9.

16. Denny, M.R. and Ratner, S.C. *Comparative Psychology: Research in Animal Behavior*, Homewood, Illinois: Dorsey Press, 1970.

17. de Boer, J.M. and Heuts, B.A. 'Prior exposure to visual cues affecting dominance in the jewel fish, *Hemichromis bimaculatus*, Gill 1862 (Pisces, Cichlidae)', *Behaviour*, 1973, *44*, pp. 299-321.

18. Figler, M.H., Dyer, R.S., Streckfus, C.F. and Nardini, K.M. 'The establishment of dominance relationships in the jewel fish, *Hemichromis bimaculatus* (Gill), as related to prior exposure to and configuration of visual cues', *Behavioral Biology*, 1975, *14*, pp. 241-5.

19. Figler, M.H., Klein, R.M. and Peeke, H.V.S. 'The establishment and reversibility of dominance relationships in jewel fish, *Hemichromis bimaculatus*, Gill (Pisces, Cichlidae): Effects of prior exposure and prior residence situations', *Behaviour*, 1976, *58*, pp. 254-71.

20. Burgett, C.A. 'Automated system for the gas–liquid chromatographic determination of acetaldehyde, ethyl acetate and fusel oils in alcoholic beverages', *Journal of the Association of Official Analytical Chemists*, 1974, *57*, pp. 1176-9.

21. Leake, C.D. and Silverman, M. *Alcoholic Beverages in Clinical Medicine*, Cleveland: The World Publishing Company, 1966.

22. Peeke, H.V.S., Cutler, L., Ellman, G., Figler, M., Gordon, D. and Peeke, S.C. 'Effects of alcohol, congeners and acetaldehyde on aggressive behavior of the convict cichlid', *Psychopharmacology*, 1981, *75*, pp. 245-7.

23. Shupe, L.M. 'Alcohol and crime. A study of the urine alcohol concentration found in 882 persons arrested during or immediately after commission of a felony', *Journal of Criminal Law and Criminology*, 1954, *44*, pp. 661-4.

24. Lagerspetz, K.M.J. 'Failure to induce aggression in mice with ethyl alcohol', *Proceedings of the International Conference on Animal Models in Alcohol Research*, (eds Eriksson, K., Kiianmaa, K. and Sinclair, J.D.), London: Academic Press, 1980, pp. 329-35.

25. Lagerspetz, K.M.J. and Ekqvist, K. 'Failure to induce aggression in inhibited and in genetically non-aggressive mice through injections of ethyl alcohol', *Aggressive Behavior*, 1978, *4*, pp. 105-13.

26. Figler, M.H. 'The hybridization of ethology and psychopharmacology in the investigation of aggressive behaviour in fish', *Multidisciplinary Approaches to Aggression Research*, (eds Brain, P.F. and Benton, D.), Amsterdam: Elsevier/North-Holland Biomedical Press, 1981, pp. 355-68.

27. Ingle, D. 'Reduction of habituation of prey-catching activity by alcohol intoxication in the frog', *Behavioral Biology*, 1973, *8*, pp. 123-9.

28. Brain, P.F. 'Differentiating types of attack and defense in rodents', *Multidisciplinary Approaches to Aggression Research* (eds Brain, P.F. and Benton, D.), Amsterdam: Elsevier/North-Holland Biomedical Press, 1981, pp. 53-78.

29. Ewart, J.P. 'Neural mechanisms of prey catching and avoidance behavior in the toad (*Bufo bufo* L.)', *Brain Behavior and Evolution*, 1970, *3*, pp. 36-54.

30. Kovach, J.K. 'Maternal behavior in the domestic cock under the influence of alcohol', *Science*, 1967, *156*, pp. 835-7.
31. Gilman, A.G., Goodman, L.S. and Gilman, A. *The Pharmacological Basis of Therapeutics*, London: MacMillan, 1980.
32. Tamimie, H.S. 'Response of alcohol treated cocks to day-old and one-week old chicks', *Poultry Science*, 1968, *47*, pp. 1366-7.
33. Meinecke, R.O. and Cherkin, A. 'Failure of ethanol or pentobarbital to suppress fighting in the pit gamecock (*Gallus gallus*)', *Psychopharmacologia*, 1972, *25*, pp. 189-94.
34. Elis, J. and Krsiak, M. 'Effect of ethanol administration during pregnancy on social behaviour of offsprings in mice', *Activitas Nervosa Superior (Praha)*, 1975, *17*, pp. 281-2.
35. Krsiak, M., Elis, J., Poschlova, N. and Masek, K. 'Increased aggressiveness and lower brain serotonin levels in offspring of mice given alcohol during gestation', *Journal of Studies on Alcohol*, 1977, *38*, pp. 1696-704.
36. Eichelman, B.S., Jr. and Thoa, N.B. 'The aggressive monoamines', *Biological Psychiatry*, 1973, *6*, pp. 143-64.
37. Branchey, L. and Friedhoff, A.J. 'The influence of ethanol administered to pregnant rats on tyrosine hydroxylase activity of their offspring', *Psychopharmacologia*, 1973, *32*, pp. 151-6.
38. Valzelli, L. '5-hydroxytryptamine in aggressiveness in *Serotonin: New Vistas, Biochemistry and Behavioural and Clinical Studies* (eds Costa, E., Gessa, G. and Sandler, M.), New York: Raven Press, 1974, pp. 255-63.
39. Goodwin, D.W., Schulsinger, F., Hermansen, L., Guze, S.B. and Winokur, G. 'Alcoholism and the hyperactive child syndrome', *Journal of Nervous and Mental Diseases*, 1975, *160*, pp. 349-53.
40. Brase, D.A. and Loh, H.H. 'Possible role of 5-hydroxytryptamine in minimal brain dysfunction', *Life Sciences*, 1975, *16*, pp. 1005-16.
41. Yanai, J. and Ginsburg, B.E. 'Long-term effects of early ethanol on predatory behaviour in inbred mice', *Physiological Psychology*, 1976, *4*, pp. 409-11.
42. Calhoun, J.B. 'Distribution and food habitats of mammals in the vicinity of the Reelfoot Lake Biological Station', *Journal of the Tennessee Academy of Science*, 1941, *16*, pp. 207-25.
43. Whitaker, J.O. 'Food of *Mus musculus, Peromyscus maniculatus bairdii* and *Peromyscus leucopus* in Vigo County, Indiana', *Journal of Mammalogy*, 1966, *47*, pp. 473-86.
44. Yanai, J., Ginsburg, B.E. and Vinopal, B. 'Comparison of early effects of ethanol on agonistic behavior in inbred strains of mice', *Behavior Genetics*, 1976, *6*, pp. 122-3.
45. Yanai, J. and Ginsburg, B.E. 'Long-term reduction of male agonistic behavior in mice following early exposure to ethanol', *Psychopharmacology*, 1977, *52*, pp. 31-4.
46. Levitsky, D.A. and Barnes, R.H. 'Nutritional and environmental interactions in the behavioral development of the rat: Long-term effects', *Science*, 1972, *176*, pp. 68-71.
47. Randt, C.T., Blizard, D.A. and Friedman, E. 'Early life undernutrition and aggression in two mice strains', *Developmental Psychobiology*, 1973, *8*, pp. 275-9.
48. Smart, J.L. 'Undernutrition and aggression', in *Multidisciplinary Approaches to Aggression Research* (eds Brain, P.F. and Benton, D.), Amsterdam: Elsevier/North-Holland Biomedical Press, 1981, pp. 179-91.
49. Dobbing, J. 'Vulnerable periods in brain growth and somatic growth' in *The Biology of Human Fetal Growth* (eds D.F. Roberts and A.M. Thompson),

London: Taylor & Francis, 1976, pp. 137-47.
50. Ewart, F.G. and Cutler, M.G. 'Effects of ethyl alcohol on development and social behaviour in the offspring of laboratory mice', *Psychopharmacology,* 1979, *62,* pp. 247-51.
51. Abel, E.L. 'Effects of ethanol on pregnant rats and their offspring', *Psychopharmacology,* 1978, *57,* pp. 5-11.
52. Anandam, N., Felegi, W. and Stern, J.M. '*In utero* alcohol heightens juvenile reactivity', *Pharmacology, Biochemistry and Behavior,* 1980, *13,* pp. 531-5.
53. Bammer, G. and Eichelman, B. 'Ethanol effects on shock-induced fighting and muricide by rats', *Aggressive Behavior,* 1983, *9,* pp. 175-81.
54. Blanchard, R.J., Blanchard, D.C. and Takahaski, L.K. 'Reflexive fighting in the albino rat: aggressive or defensive behavior?', *Aggressive Behavior,* 1977, *3,* pp. 145-55.
55. Brain, P.F. *Hormones, Drugs and Aggression, Vol. 3,* Annual Research Reviews, Montreal: Eden Press, 1979.
56. Blanchard, R.J. and Blanchard, D.C. 'Aggressive behavior in rats', *Behavioral Biology,* 1977, *21,* pp. 197-224.
57. Moyer, K.E. 'Kinds of aggression and their physiological basis', *Communications in Behavioral Biology,* 1968, *2,* pp. 65-87.
58. Brain, P.F., Al-Maliki, S. and Benton, D. 'Attempts to determine the status of electroshock-induced attack in laboratory mice', *Behavioural Processes,* 1981, *6,* pp. 171-89.
59. Pohorecky, L.A. 'Biphasic action of ethanol', *Biobehavioral Reviews,* 1977, *1,* pp. 231-40.
60. Irwin, S., Kinohi, R., Van Sloten, M. and Workman, M.P. 'Drug effects on distress-evoked behavior in mice: methodology and drug class comparisons', *Psychopharmacologia,* 1971, *20,* pp. 172-85.
61. Weitz, M.K. 'Effects of ethanol on shock-elicited fighting behavior in rats', *Quarterly Journal of Studies on Alcohol,* 1974, *35,* pp. 953-8.
62. Schaaf, T.G. 'The effects of alcohol on pain-elicited aggression', *M.S. thesis,* Eastern Washington State College, 1971.
63. Tramill, J.L., Wesley, A.L. and Davis, S.F. 'The effects of chronic ethanol challenges on aggressive responding in rats maintained on a semideprivation diet', *Bulletin of the Psychonomic Society,* 1981, *17,* pp. 51-2.
64. Tramill, J.L., Gustavson, K., Weaver, M.S., Moore, S.A. and Davis, S.F. 'Shock-elicited aggression as a function of acute and chronic ethanol challenges', *The Journal of General Psychology,* 1983, *109,* pp. 53-8.
65. Azrin, N.H., Rubin, H.B. and Hutchinson, R.R. 'Biting attack by rats in response to aversive shock', *Journal of the Experimental Analysis of Behavior,* 1968, *11,* pp. 633-9.
66. Wagner, G.C., Beuving, L.J. and Hutchinson, R.R. 'Androgen-dependency of aggressive target-biting and paired fighting in male mice', *Physiology and Behavior,* 1979, *22,* pp. 43-6.
67. Brain, P.F., Al-Maliki, S., Parmigiani, S. and Hammour, H.A. 'Studies on tube restraint-induced attack on a metal target by laboratory mice', *Behavioural Processes,* 1983, *8,* pp. 277-87.
68. Wagner, G.C., Beuving, L.J. and Hutchinson, R.R. 'The effects of gonadal hormone manipulations on aggressive target-biting in mice', *Aggressive Behavior,* 1980, *6,* pp. 1-7.
69. Tramill, J.L., Turner, P.E., Sisemore, D.A. and Davis, S.F. Hungry, drunk, and not real mad: the effects of alcohol injections on aggressive responding', *Bulletin of the Psychonomic Society,* 1980, *15,* pp. 339-41.
70. Smoothy, R. and Berry, M.S. 'Effects of ethanol on murine aggression

assessed by biting of an inanimate target', *Psychopharmacology*, 1984, *83*, pp. 268-71.

71. Al-Hazmi, M. and Brain, P.F. 'Effects of age, habituation and alcohol administration on tube restraint-induced attack by Swiss mice', *Aggressive Behavior*, 1984, 10, p. 145.

72. Smoothy, R. 'Videotape analysis of the effect of alcohol on aggressive and other behaviour in laboratory mice (*Mus musculus* L.)', PhD thesis, University of Wales, 1985.

73. Krsiak, M. and Borgesova, M. 'Drugs and spontaneous behaviour: why are detailed studies still so rare?' *Activitas Nervosa Superior (Praha)*, 1972, *14*, pp. 285-93.

74. Borgesova, M., Kadlecova, O. and Krsiak, M. 'Behaviour of untreated mice to alcohol- or chlordiazepoxide-treated partners', *Activitas Nervosa Superior (Praha)*, 1971, *13*, pp. 206-7.

75. Yoshimura, H. and Ogawa, N. 'Pharmaco-ethological analysis of agonistic behavior between resident and intruder mice: effects of ethyl alcohol', *Folia pharmacologica*, Japan, 1983, *81*, pp. 135-41.

76. Miczek, K.A., Winslow, J.T. and DeBold, J.F. 'Heightened aggressive behavior by animals interacting with alcohol-treated conspecifics: studies with mice, rats and squirrel monkeys', *Pharmacology, Biochemistry and Behavior*, 1984, *20*, pp. 349-53.

77. Krsiak, M. and Borgesova, M. 'Effect of alcohol on behaviour of pairs of rats', *Psychopharmacologia*, 1973, *32*, pp. 201-9.

78. Borgesova, M. and Krsiak, M. 'Effect of alcohol on a dyadic interaction in rats', *Activitas Nervosa Superior (Praha)*, 1972, *14*, pp. 168-9.

79. Silverman, A.P. 'Behaviour of rats given a "smoking dose" of nicotine', *Animal Behaviour*, 1971, *19*, pp. 67-74.

80. Grant, E.C. and Mackintosh, J.H. 'A comparison of the social postures of some common laboratory rodents', *Behaviour*, 1963, *21*, pp. 246-59.

81. Chance, M.R.A., Mackintosh, J.H. and Dixon, A.K. 'The effects of ethyl alcohol on social encounters between mice', *Journal of Alcoholism*, 1973, *8*, pp. 90-3.

82. Krsiak, M. 'Effect of ethanol on aggression and timidity in mice', *Psychopharmacology*, 1976, *51*, pp. 75-80.

83. Krsiak, M. 'Timid singly-housed mice: their value in prediction of psychotropic activity of drugs', *British Journal of Pharmacology*, 1975, *35*, pp. 141-50.

84. Mettala, R. 'A factorial study of the behavior of mice in simulation experiments eliciting aggressive responses', *Reports from the Institute of Psychology, University of Turku*, 1965, *15*, pp. 1-7.

85. Miczek, K.A. and Barry, H. III 'Effects of alcohol on attack and defensive-submissive reactions in rats', *Psychopharmacology*, 1977, *52*, pp. 231-7.

86. Miczek, K.A. and O'Donnell, J.M. 'Alcohol and chlordiazepoxide increase suppressed aggression in mice', *Psychopharmacology*, 1980, *69*, pp. 39-44.

87. Smoothy, R. and Berry, M.S. 'Effects of alcohol on different models of rodent aggression', *Aggressive Behavior*, 1984, 10, pp. 172-3.

88. Smoothy, R., Berry, M.S. and Brain, P.F. 'Influences of alcohol on the social responses of male resident mice to anosmic female intruders', *Behavioural Processes*, 1985, in press.

89. Mackintosh, J.H. 'Territory formation by laboratory mice', *Animal Behaviour*, 1970, *18*, pp. 177-83.

90. Dixon, A.K. and Mackintosh, J.H. 'Effects of female urine upon the social behaviour of adult male mice', *Animal Behaviour*, 1971, *19*, pp. 138-140.

91. Bertilson, H.S., Mead, J.D., Morgret, M.K. and Dengerink, H.A. 'Measurement of mouse squeals for 23 hours as evidence of long-term effects of alcohol on aggression in pairs of mice', *Psychological Reports*, 1977, *41*, pp. 247-50.

92. Morgret, M.K. 'An apparatus for detection and counting of mouse squeals', *Behavior Research Methods and Instrumentation*, 1972, *4*, pp. 21-3.

93. Morgret, M.K. and Dengerink, H.A. 'The squeal as an indicator of aggression in mice', *Behavior Research Methods and Instrumentation*, 1972, *4*, pp. 138-40.

94. Miczek, K.A. and DeBold, J.F. 'Hormone-drug interactions and their influence on aggressive behavior' in *Hormones and Aggressive Behavior* (ed B. Svare), New York: Plenum Press, 1983, pp. 313-47.

95. Smoothy, R. and Berry, M.S. 'Ethanol and social behaviour in naîve Swiss mice', *Aggressive Behavior*, 1982, *8*, pp. 204-7.

96. Alberts, J.R. 'Producing and interpreting experimental olfactory deficits', *Physiology and Behavior*, 1974, *12*, pp. 657-70.

97. Brain, P.F. and Al-Maliki, S. 'A comparison of "intermale fighting" in "standard opponent" tests and attack directed towards locusts by "TO" strain mice: effects of simple experimental manipulations', *Animal Behaviour*, 1978, *26*, pp. 723-37.

98. Smoothy, R. and Berry, M.S. 'Effects of ethanol on behaviour of aggressive mice from two different strains: a comparison of simple and complex behavioural assessments', *Pharmacology, Biochemistry and Behavior*, 1983, *19*, pp. 645-53.

99. Smoothy, R., Berry, M.S. and Brain, P.F. 'Acute influences of ethanol on murine social aggression: effects of dose, strain and fighting experience', *Aggressive Behavior*, 1983, *9*, pp. 119-20.

100. Lagerspetz, K.M.J. 'Studies on the aggressive behaviour of mice', *Annales de l'Academie des Sciences Fennicae, Series B*, 1964, *131/3*, pp. 1-131.

101. Arvola, A. 'A method for recording general activity of mice', *Acta Physiologica Scandinavica*, 1960, *49*, pp. 62-4.

102. Goldsmith, J.F., Brain, P.F. and Benton, D. 'Effects of age at differential housing and the duration of individual housing/grouping on intermale fighting behavior and adrenocortical activity in "TO" strain mice', *Aggressive Behavior*, 1976, *2*, pp. 307-23.

103. Miczek, K.A. and Barry, H. III 'Pharmacology of sex and aggression' in *Behavioral Pharmacology* (eds Glick, S.D. and Goldfarb, D.), St Louis: C.V. Mosby Press, 1976, pp. 176-257.

104. Miczek, K.A. and Krsiak, M. 'Drug effects on agonistic behavior' in *Advances in Behavioral Pharmacology (Vol. 2)* (eds Thompson, T. and Dews, P.B.), New York: Academic Press, 1979, pp. 87-162.

105. Brain, P.F., Benton, D., Childs, G. and Parmigiani, S. 'The effect of the type of opponent in tests of murine aggression', *Behavioural Processes*, 1981, *6*, pp. 319-27.

106. Parmigiani, S. and Brain, P.F. 'Effects of residence, aggressive experience and intruder familiarity on attack shown by male mice', *Behavioural Processes*, 1983, *8*, pp. 45-57.

107. Smoothy, R. and Berry, M.S. 'Alcohol increases both locomotion and immobility in mice: an ethological analysis of spontaneous locomotor activity', *Psychopharmacology*, 1984, *83*, pp. 272-6.

108. Bloom, F., Lad, P., Pittman, Q. and Rogers, J. 'Blood alcohol levels in rats: non-uniform yields from intraperitoneal doses based on body weight', *British Journal of Pharmacology*, 1982, *75*, pp. 251-4.

109. Thompson, T. and Schuster, C.R. *Behavioral Pharmacology*, New

Jersey: Prentice-Hall Inc., 1968.

110. Cutler, M.G., Mackintosh, J.H. and Chance, M.R.A. 'Effects of the environment on the behavioural response of mice to non-ataxic doses of ethyl alcohol', *Neuropharmacology*, 1975, *14*, pp. 841-6.

111. Cutler, M.G. 'Changes in the social behaviour of laboratory mice during administration and on withdrawal from non-ataxic doses of ethyl alcohol', *Neuropharmacology*, 1976, *15*, pp. 495-8.

112. Freund, G. 'Alcohol withdrawal syndrome in mice', *Archives of Neurology*, 1969, *21*, pp. 315-20.

113. Masserman, J.H. and Jacobson, L. 'Effects of ethyl alcohol on the cerebral cortex and the hypothalamus of the cat', *Archives of Neurology and Psychiatry*, 1940, *43*, pp. 334-40.

114. Masserman, J.H. 'Drugs, brain and behaviour: an experimental approach to experiential psychoses', *Journal of Neuropsychiatry*, 1962, *3*, S104-S113.

115. Woodworth, R.S. and Sherrington, C.S. 'A pseudoactive reflex and its spinal path', *Journal of Physiology*, 1904, *31*, pp. 234-43.

116. Wasman, M. and Flynn, J.P. 'Directed attack elicited from the hypothalamus', *Archives of Neurology*, 1962, *6*, pp. 220-7.

117. Flynn, J.P. 'Patterning mechanisms, patterned reflexes, and attack behavior in cats', *Nebraska Symposium on Motivation* (eds Cole, J.K. and Jensen, D.D.), Lincoln: University of Nebraska Press, 1972, pp. 125-53.

118. MacDonnell, M.F. and Ehmer, M, 'Some effects of ethanol on aggressive behavior in cats', *Quarterly Journal of Studies on Alcohol*, 1969, *30*, pp. 312-19.

119. MacDonnell, M.F. and Fessock, L. 'Some effects of ethanol, amphetamine, disulfiram and p-CPA on seizing of prey in feline predatory attack and on associated motor pathways', *Quarterly Journal of Studies on Alcohol*, 1972, *33*, pp. 437-50.

120. Kabat, H., Anson, J.B., Magoun, H.W. and Ranson, S.W. 'Stimulation of the hypothalamus, with special reference to its effect on gastrointestinal motility', *American Journal of Physiology*, 1935, *112*, pp. 214-26.

121. Hess, W.R. and Brugger, M. 'Das subkortikale Zentrum der affektiven Abwehrreaktion', *Helvetica Physiologica and Pharmacologica Acta*, 1943, *1*, pp. 35-52.

122. MacDonnell, M.F., Fessock, L. and Brown, S.H. 'Ethanol and the neural substrate for affective defense in the cat', *Quarterly Journal of Studies on Alcohol*, 1971, *32*, pp. 406-19.

123. Ruusunen, S., Johansson, G., Huhtala, A., Niskanen, H. and Paakkonen, T. 'Ethyl alcohol and defence behaviour in the cat', *Medical Biology*, 1975, *53*, pp. 475-80.

124. Johansson, G.G. 'Neural stimulation as a means of generating standardized threat under laboratory conditions' in *Multidisciplinary Approaches to Aggression Research* (eds Brain, P.F. and Benton, D.), Amsterdam: Elsevier/North-Holland Biomedical Press, 1981, pp. 93-100.

125. James, W.T, 'The effect of the presence of a second individual on the conditioned salivary response in dogs of different constitutional types', *Journal of Genetic Psychology*, 1936, *49*, pp. 437-49.

126. James, W.T. 'Further experiments in social behavior among dogs', *Journal of Genetic Psychology*, 1939, *54*, pp. 151-64.

127. Scott, J.P. *Aggression*, Chicago–London: University of Chicago Press, 1975.

128. James, W.T. 'Dominant and submissive behavior in puppies as indicated by food intake', *Journal of Genetic Psychology*, 1949, *75*, pp. 33-43.

129. Pettijohn, T.F. 'The effects of alcohol on agonistic behavior in the Telomian dog', *Psychopharmacology*, 1979, *60*, pp. 295-301.

130. Scott, J.P., Elliot, O., Trattner, A. and Kirshenbaum, J. 'A note on Telomian dogs: an aboriginal breed from Malaysia', *Carnivore Genetics Newsletter*, 1967, *3*, pp. 45-8.
131. Scott, J.P. and Fuller, J.L. *Genetics and the Social Behavior of the Dog*, Chicago–London: University of Chicago Press, 1965.
132. Bernstein, I.S. and Mason, W.A. 'Activity patterns of rhesus monkeys in a social group', *Animal Behaviour*, 1963, *11*, pp. 455-60.
133. Plotnick, R.J., King, F. and Roberts, L. 'An objective analysis of social dominance in the squirrel monkey', *Proceedings of the 73rd Annual Convention of the American Psychological Association*, 1965, pp. 109-19.
134. Varley, M. and Symmes, D. 'The hierarchy of dominance in a group of macaques', *Behaviour*, 1966, *27*, pp. 54-75.
135. Stahl, W.R. and Malinow, M.R. 'A survey of physiological measurements in *Macaca mulatta*', *Folia Primatologica*, 1967, *7*, pp. 12-33.
136. Cressman, R.J. and Cadell, T.E. 'Drinking and the social behavior of rhesus monkeys', *Quarterly Journal of Studies on Alcohol*, 1971, *32*, pp. 764-74.
137. Peretti, P.O. and Lewis, B.R. 'Affects of alcoholic consumption on the activity patterns of individual rhesus monkeys and their behavior in a social group', *Primates*, 1969, *10*, pp. 181-8.
138. Maslow, A.H. 'The role of dominance in the social and sexual behavior of infra-human primates. I. Observations at Vilas Park Zoo', *Journal of General Psychology*, 1936, *48*, pp. 261-77.
139. Crowley, J.T., Stynes, A.J., Hydinger, M. and Kaufman, C. 'Ethanol, methamphetamine, pentobarbital, morphine, and monkey social behavior', *Archives of General Psychiatry*, 1974, *31*, pp. 829-38.
140. Kaufman, I.C. and Rosenblum, L. 'A behavioral taxonomy for *Macaca nemestrina* and *Macaca radiata*', *Primates*, 1966, *7*, pp. 205-58.
141. MacAndrew, C. and Edgerton, R.E. *Drunken Comportment*, Chicago: Aldine, 1969, p. 197.
142. Chamove, A.S. and Harlow, H.F. 'Exaggeration of self-aggression following alcohol ingestion in rhesus monkeys', *Journal of Abnormal Psychology*, 1970, *75*, pp. 207-9.
143. Tinklepaugh, O.L. 'The self-mutilation of a male macacus rhesus monkey', *Journal of Mammology*, 1928, *9*, pp. 293-300.
144. Cross, H.A. and Harlow, H.F. 'Prolonged and progressive effects of partial isolation on the behaviour of macaque monkeys', *Journal of Experimental Research in Personality*, 1965, *1*, pp. 39-49.
145. Kamback, M.C. 'Alcohol selection, learning performance, and emotionality in two subspecies of monkeys (*Macaca nemestrina*)', *Proceedings of the 80th Annual Convention of the American Psychological Association*, 1972, pp. 841-2.
146. Butters, C.M., Mishkin, M. and Minsky, A.F. 'Emotional responses toward humans in monkeys with selective frontal lesions', *Physiology and Behavior*, 1968, *3*, pp. 213-15.
147. Kamback, M.C. 'The effects of orbital and dorsolateral frontal cortical ablations on ethanol self-selection and emotional behaviors in monkeys (*Macaca nemestrina*)', *Neuropsychologia*, 1973, *11*, pp. 331-5.
148. Butters, C.M., Snyder, D.R. and McDonald, J.A. 'Effects of orbitofrontal lesions on aversive and aggressive behaviors in rhesus monkeys', *Journal of Comparative and Physiological Psychology*, 1970, *72*, pp. 132-44.
149. Carpentier, J.A. and Armenti, N.P. 'Some behavioral effects of alcohol on man' in *The Biology of Alcoholism, Vol. II* (eds Kissin, B. and Begleiter, H.), New York: Plenum Press, 1972.
150. Hinde, R. *Biological Bases of Human Social Behavior*, New York:

McGraw-Hill Book Company, 1974.

151. Brain, P.F. 'Human aggression and the physical environment' in *Mental Health and the Human Environment* (ed. Freeman, H.L.), London: Churchill-Livingstone, 1984, pp. 97-120.

152. Brain, P.F. 'Comments on laboratory-based "aggression" tests', *Animal Behaviour*, 1984, *32*, pp. 1256-7.

5 ALCOHOL AND VIOLENCE: PROBLEMS RELATING TO METHODOLOGY, STATISTICS AND CAUSATION

Charles M. Evans

Introduction

Many studies have linked alcohol consumption with a variety of violent acts. Some authors find 'alcoholics' over-represented in statistics on violent behaviour, whilst others have suggested that many individuals (whether alcoholic or not) had consumed alcohol shortly before committing acts of violence. Types of violent behaviour reviewed in these studies include felony,[1,2] criminal homicide,[3,4] violence within the family,[5,6] sexual assault,[7,8,9] (see also Chapter 6), suicide[10,11] and various types of violent accident.[12,13] There is also some evidence that a high proportion of victims had been drinking before being robbed or physically assaulted, suggesting that intoxication made such individuals more vulnerable to attack[3,14] (See also Chapter 6). It is consequently of no surprise that authorities have expressed concern and that many research groups have directed considerable effort towards gaining an understanding of the relationship between alcohol ingestion and violence.

This chapter extends previous work[15,16] by exploring the complex statistical link between this drug and behaviour. This analysis will briefly summarise the literature on the varieties of violence mentioned above. The methods used to obtain such data will then be critically examined and problems associated with their interpretation explored. The idea that there is a causal link between alcohol and violence will be considered, and the implications for the medical, psychological and social treatment of violent offenders will be examined.

Data Linking Alcohol Ingestion and/or Alcoholism with Violence

Violence (as noted in Chapter 1) is a word that can be used as a convenient label linking a wide range of human activities and events which can be characterised by great physical force, impetuosity, passion or simply injury to individuals. There are clearly many different kinds of 'violence', but it seems convenient to embrace a wide definition of these phenomena in order to draw attention to the potential range of harmful consequences of alcohol consumption. The reader should not assume that the drawing together of such data suggests that these phenomena have a common causal basis, or that alcohol influences them in the same way. It should also be emphasised that information from the studies forming the basis of the following section is presented without commenting on its scientific validity. Later sections provide a detailed analysis of the statistical and methodological problems associated with such data.

Petty Crime, Felony and Homicide

The consumption of alcohol and a presumed elevated blood-alcohol concentration (BAC) have been linked with petty crime, home quarrels and minor out-breaks of public disorder.[17,18,19] In a study of delinquency, 63 per cent of prisoners in a young offender's institution in Scotland claimed to have been intoxicated when committing the crime for which they had been imprisoned.[20] A large proportion of homicides and other violent crimes also reportedly involved the offender drinking shortly before the incidents took place.[1,3,21,22,23] The rates vary between different localities and countries, but wherever alcohol is freely available, often more than 30 per cent and sometimes as many as 77 per cent of the individuals accused of murder have been presumed to have been drinking before the offence.[24] For instance, one well-documented study[25] revealed that between 1953 and 1974, 58 per cent of the 365 men accused of murder in the West of Scotland were intoxicated at the time of their offence. Many of these offences occurred on a Friday evening, at weekends or on public holidays, when alcohol consumption is likely to be maximal.[26,27]

Violent offences tend to be more frequently associated with drinking than do non-violent ones; and alcohol-related crimes are less likely to be premeditated than acts that do not involve this drug.[28] The more violent assaults are frequently carried out with knives or sharp instruments.[1,29] In many cases the victim had been drinking before being assaulted, robbed or murdered. For example, Gillies[25] reported that 42 per cent of victims drank before being murdered. This finding is typical of a number of other studies,[6,24,29] and has given rise to the concept of the 'battered alcoholic syndrome'.[14] In some cases the victims, who are generally male,[29] may be simply made more vulnerable to attack by their intoxication, but in other examples the victims appear to have initiated the violence.[3,29]

As well as finding that many individuals drink shortly before committing acts of violence, a high rate of alcoholism among individuals convicted of criminal acts is evident. The reports vary, but in a series of studies in the USA, alcoholism among convicted felons has been reported in 17-48 per cent of cases,[4,30,31,32] a rate much higher than the general population where 5-10 per cent[33] are alcoholics. Studies in the United Kingdom yield similar results.[28,34,35] Despite this evidence, there is no simple correlation between alcohol consumption and homicide when these are compared over a range of countries in Europe or even in different states of the USA.[36] This is partly because national and local traditions have a strong influence on the prevalence of alcohol-related problems, regardless of the precise level of *per capita* consumption.[37] In some countries drunkenness rarely leads to violence,[38] whereas in Iceland 77 per cent of incidents are reported to involve alcohol, although the homicide rate in this country is remarkably low compared to neighbouring Greenland.[24]

Sexual Assault

Recent studies have reported that alcohol was consumed by a high proportion (30-50 per cent) of rapists shortly before their assaults.[1,8,39,40] A high rate of alcoholism has also been noted in convicted rapists.[40] Unfortunately, researchers in this field often consider rape in isolation from other sex crimes — a seemingly arbitrary distinction. As Coid (Chapter 6 in this volume) thoroughly reviews the area of alcohol, rape and sexual assault, little more will be said here.

As with other forms of crime, there may be an association between rapes occurring at the weekend and the ingestion of alcohol. According to one study,[39] alcohol consumption was linked with 40 per cent of the 344 rapes committed on Fridays, Saturdays and Sundays, but to 28 per cent of the 302 rapes committed on weekdays.

Violence Within the Family

It has been reported that violence is more than twice as likely to occur in families with alcohol-related problems.[6] The violence is usually directed towards the wife, but assaults on children are also frequent.[6,41] One study indicated that, of all marital assaults reported to the police, half occurred after the husband had been drinking.[42] Gayford[41] reported a similar proportion of alcohol-related assault by husbands of women seeking aid at a refuge or in general psychiatric consultation.

A smaller proportion of women also admit to drunkenness on more than the isolated occasion.[41] Not only may children be assaulted by their fathers following a drinking bout, but 37 per cent of women in Gayford's study admitted 'explosive outbursts' with their children especially after they themselves had been subjected to violence. Some children were also assaulted when trying to intervene when their father was being violent towards their mother.

It may seem surprising but it has been found that women battered by alcohol-abusing husbands tend to carry the conditions of their early family situation into marriage. Many women who had had violent, alcohol-abusing fathers lived with or married men knowing that they drank heavily and could be violent.[5] In some cases, after such a relationship has broken down, the women might enter a second or a third such relationship.[43] The reasons for these findings are obscure, but it has been suggested that the social and environmental circumstances of such women favour contact with men who drink heavily and have a tendency for violence, rather than being expressions of the woman's choice.[43]

Suicide

There are many studies which link the consumption of alcohol and/or alcoholism with suicide or attempted suicide. Goodwin[4] found that a quarter of all suicide victims, whether or not alcoholic, drank shortly before death; and several studies have reported a raised post-mortem BAC (0.05 per cent or over) in 30 per cent or more of successful suicides. Other studies show that individuals frequently drink prior to self-injury or unsuccessful suicide attempts.[10,44,45,46]

It also appears that a high proportion of successful suicide victims were alcoholics.[47,48] Alcoholism is also more common amongst attempted suicides,[49,50] and suicidal behaviour (completed, attempted or contemplated) occurs more frequently in alcoholics than in the general population.[49,50,51]

Accidental Injury

Consumption of alcohol or a diagnosis of alcoholism has been linked with accidental injury or death resulting from drowning,[52] fire,[12] falling,[53] aircraft crashes,[54] and dangers associated with the workplace.[55] Although individuals may be accidentally killed or injured in the most violent circumstances, there is no evidence of aggressive intent because the incidents are classed as accidents. Obviously, some 'accidents' could have been successful suicides or even murders, and it is possible that certain driving 'accidents' result from 'sub-conscious' aggressive or self-destructive impulses.[13] In general, this type of violence appears differently motivated from the earlier-described categories.

Problems in the Interpretation of Statistics

Despite the seemingly overwhelming body of literature presented above, many authors refrain from expressing unequivocal views about a causal relationship between alcohol and violence. This is not necessarily because the association cannot be analysed, but simply reflects the belief that the consumption of alcohol may be misreported due to bias in the method of data collection. The varied ways in which this can happen are discussed below.

Differences Between Studies

Myers[28] has suggested that many authors are disturbed by differences between studies in the rates of reported alcohol consumption, the occasions on which such drinking is associated with violence and differences between accounts of the assailant's pattern of habitual drinking. As indicated earlier, much of this variability may be related to differences between societies or social groups in terms of traditional levels of alcohol consumption and attitudes to violence, but there are also considerable variations in data sources. For example, evidence may come from studies of prison and other custodial populations or psychiatric patients, and the actual data may be supplied by medical workers, laboratory-based scientists, the police, court reports or even by self-reports. Another source of variation is the set of criteria used to define 'alcoholism' or 'problem' drinking' in different studies.

Methods of Expressing Rates of Association

Many studies report the proportion of the studied population who drank shortly before committing an offence, or the proportion who were alcoholic without comparison with a suitable control group or even with reference to the general populace. Statistics presented in this way invariably exaggerate the association between alcohol and behaviour. For example, the rate of alcoholism in the general population may be as much as 10 per cent[33,56] so that the rate found in a group of violent individuals must be well above that to suggest a significant relationship. Even comparisons with the general population may be misleading since different socio-economic groups may differ on this measure.[57] It is therefore desirable that a suitably matched control be selected for comparison wherever possible.

Data linking violence with prior acute consumption presents an even greater problem. A rate of 30 per cent of alcohol-related offences would be of no significance if it merely reflected the proportion of that sex and social grouping which might be expected to have a raised BAC at similar times. This estimation is rarely considered.

It is interesting to re-examine the data relating to the incidence of murder in the West of Scotland between 1953 and 1974[24] in the light of the above comments. Saunders and Kershaw[58] have examined the prevalence of problem drinking in this area and, although their data refer to more recent times, report that 67 per cent of males in this region classified themselves as 'regular drinkers' and consumed an average of 20 units of alcohol per week (equivalent to 10 pints (5.7 l) of beer or 20 fl. oz (0.57 l) of spirits). As mentioned earlier, much of this drinking occurs on Fridays and at the weekend when most murders are likely to be committed.[25,26] Consequently, it is probable that at these times a high percentage of males in the general population of this region will have a raised BAC. The high rate of alcohol-associated murders may partially reflect this background figure rather than a causal relationship between alcohol and murder.

It is difficult to assess the extent to which data relating alcohol and violence can be misleading. It seems unlikely, however, that the statistics can be wholly discredited. Alcoholics still seem over-represented in violent sub-groups when compared to the general population.[56,59] Moreover, in a well-constructed study, Myers[27] showed that violent criminals were more likely to have consumed alcohol shortly before committing the offence for which they were imprisoned than were non-violent counterparts. These two sub-groups were similar on 25 biographical variables including education, place of birth, occupation, income, area of residence and numbers of children.

Self-reports of Alcohol Consumption and BAC

Many studies listed above rely heavily on self-reports of alcohol consumption as a basis for their statistics. There is naturally some scepticism concerning their validity although some studies do indicate that self-reports may be relatively reliable in many circumstances.[60,61,62] However, a defendant may report or exaggerate the use of alcohol as an excuse for his behaviour,[63,64] even though drunkenness is no defence in most legal systems.[65,66]

Another source of bias might arise when the victim of an assault mentions to the police that he or she was drinking before the incident. The credibility of such victims may be reduced such that there is some doubt as to where the incident took place, the identity of the assailant, or even if the assault took place.[67] In such cases the police may be reluctant to press charges in the face of potentially insufficient or doubtful evidence. This phenomenon may be of greatest significance in cases of rape, since the defence frequently does not dispute that intercourse has taken place, but suggests that the victim had consented. In the absence of corroborative evidence (such as physical injury), a jury may also be reluctant to convict of rape,[68] especially if they believe that the victim was intoxicated at the time and perhaps less likely to resist sexual advances.[69] There may also be a tendency for victims to avoid mentioning that they had been drinking, in an attempt to avoid some of these problems.

Direct BAC measurement might appear better evidence of drinking than self-reports, but even this type of data can seriously mislead. First, it is not feasible to measure BAC in most cases as the assailant is likely to be apprehended some time after the assault has taken place. Secondly, convicted assailants may not be representative of all offenders with respect to their use of alcohol. It has been estimated that three-fifths of violent criminals are not identified by the police, meaning that it is quite possible that statistics presented in most cases refer to 'bungled' crime.[64] This suggests that the high rate of association between raised BAC and violent crime, rather than supporting a causal relationship, reveals that intoxication makes it less likely that individual participants will escape detection. This notion of 'alcohol-related bungling' is supported by data indicating that many violent crimes associated with alcohol tend to be spontaneous and poorly planned.[27]

The Police and the Legal System

There are a number of ways in which bias can be introduced into the analysis when data are obtained from incidents which have been processed by the police and the legal system. As mentioned earlier, the involvement of alcohol may render an assailant more likely to be caught by the police; and victims who admit that they had been drinking may find it difficult to establish their credibility.

Other stages of the legal process introduce further opportunities for the statistics to be distorted. A study by Baldwin and McConville[70] on 121 cases in Birmingham Crown Court (England) involved a variety of alleged offences including burglary, rape and unlawful wounding. Seventy per cent of defendants pleaded guilty because of pressure from their own barristers, or because they had been involved in some negotiation which resulted in a plea of guilty to a lesser charge being associated with a shorter sentence. In one case, a man with a previous history of violence had been involved in a fight at a dance. He was charged with 'wounding with intent' since his victim had sustained serious injury when the defendant had hit him with a glass vase. He was also charged with 'criminal damage' for breaking the vase, and after plea bargaining the prosecution accepted a plea of guilty to this crime but not guilty to wounding with intent. The man was fined, and told the investigators that he couldn't believe his luck. Another case involved a young man with previous convictions for sexual offences who was initially charged with rape. There was clear evidence of sexual intercourse and good reason to believe that the victim had not consented. In order to spare an immature girl the ordeal of giving evidence in court, the prosecution agreed to a plea of guilty to the lesser charge of 'indecent assault'. This assailant was also fined and said later 'Had I not been told by the barrister, I might have pleaded guilty to rape.'

It is beyond the scope of this chapter to consider the implications of cases such as the above for the legal system, but the impact of such decision-making on assessing the association between alcohol and violence must be commented upon. It is likely that the first case described here involved alcohol but, for reasons of legal convenience, it did not find its way into statistics relating to violent assault. The second case illustrates one of the many reasons why rape has the lowest conviction rate of all violent crimes, and how a case which should enter the statistics on such offences is channelled into a group of lesser offences. There seems no way, at the present time, of assessing the impact of this filtering effect on the frequency of prosecuted rape cases involving alcohol.

The 'Causal' Link Between Alcohol and Violence

In trying to persuade the reader that there is a link between alcohol and violence, a writer may over-state his case. Since the role of a scientist is to express the data fairly and to make inferences with as much objectivity as is humanly possible, we should perhaps start by placing this phenomenon in a correct perspective. Clearly, in all the types of violence referred to earlier, alcohol or alcoholism was generally involved only in a minority of cases. If the background figures on alcoholism in the general population or the numbers of individuals who are likely to have a raised BAC are taken into account, the significance of these data is still further reduced. Alcohol is obviously just one of a number of 'causes' of violence, along with social and situational determinants. If this drug did not exist, there are many other reasons why humans would continue to behave violently towards each other.

Alcohol-related violence is rare in relation to the number of man-hours devoted to drinking. For example, one study[71] showed that in 633 hours of observation in 185 bars in Vancouver, revealed *no* incidents which involved brawls or physical injury. It is true, nevertheless, that crime and violence continue to cause concern in civilised societies such that any insight into its causation must be considered important.

There appears to be two different kinds of link between alcohol and violence. When alcohol is initially consumed, an acute pharmacological effect on behaviour is recorded, but there is also a link between chronic alcohol abuse and violence which is presumed to be unrelated to the acute intoxicating effects of this drug (these phenomena are discussed in detail in Chapter 3). It is convenient to consider these associations separately.

Acute Pharmacological Effects of Alcohol

It is quite common for reviews on alcohol and violence to group together data on accidents, suicide, homicide etc. without commenting on motivation or causation. The reader may be left to assume that all these acts share a common cause, i.e. the potentiation of 'aggression' by alcohol.[72,73] Can alcohol-related violent behaviour generally be accounted for by a pharmacologically induced increase in 'aggressiveness'? Several authors favour the hypothesis that alcohol in some way generates, aggressive tendencies[3,72,73,74] whilst others support the 'disinhibition' theory.[34,75,76] The latter concept involves the belief that man has latent aggressive tendencies which are generally kept in check by 'higher neural centres' or the 'super-ego'. Alcohol is said to impair the inhibitions, 'allowing' the aggression to appear. This emotion is usually directed towards other individuals, but some authors believe that self-directed motivation may result in depression or suicide.[77,78,79]

It is important to realise that our current knowledge of the neural mechanisms 'governing' behaviour is less than precise (see Chapter 2). Entities such as 'aggressive tendencies' or 'super-ego mechanism' have yet to be translated into measurable physiological processes. It may be that alcohol can reduce inhibitions or generate aggressive motivation, but the experimental data suggest that these are likely to be general effects on behaviour, rather than specific actions on the neural centres controlling 'aggression'. Even experiments with 'simple' infra-human animals do not reveal a clear causal relationship between alcohol treatment and aggression (see Chapter 4).

In the human situation, some individuals become aggressive; some become talkative and others amorous or tearful after alcohol exposure, depending on the personality and the social situation.[80,81,82,83] The study by Grayham, La Rocque, Yetman, Ross and Guistra[71] showed that the rate of aggressive incidents (e.g. insults, gestures and mild physical aggression) was predictable in a number of bar-rooms in Vancouver on the basis of social and environmental variables. Although little aggression is seen in establishments with a friendly atmosphere, suburban location, good decor and efficient ventilation, much more is seen in less pleasant establishments. Perhaps the more violent or anti-social individuals gravitate to the poorest bars, but subjects may also tend to behave according to the expected norm for that social environment. As mentioned earlier, drunkenness rarely leads to violence in some cultures, whilst in others alcohol may be associated with a high proportion of aggressive incidents. Clearly, Carpentier and Armenti's statement[83] that 'the circumstances of drinking produce greater changes in behaviour than the alcohol does' seems very relevant.

Although alcohol is likely to promote the occurrence of behaviour most appropriate for a given circumstance, one should not dismiss the possibility that certain individuals (because they have a pathological personality or have learned to behave in an antisocial way) react to a given situation in ways judged by others to be inappropriate and that alcohol enhances such behaviour. Perception by the intoxicated individual of what is acceptable behaviour may also be impaired, leading to clearly inappropriate actions.

In the laboratory it has been shown that individuals who have ingested alcohol are more willing to administer electric shocks to others[74,75,84] Lang, Goeckner, Adesso, and Marlett[85] found that the expectation of the effects of alcohol, rather than the drug itself, potentiated shock-giving in the above context. For example, subjects who had been told that they had received alcohol but had actually received flavoured placebo, were more 'aggressive' on this measure than counterparts receiving alcohol who had been told that they were drinking placebo.

It should not be assumed that the motivational control of shock-giving and that of violent crime are the same although such an assumption is often inherent in the first-mentioned type of study. These experiments do, however, highlight the power of suggestion which may outweigh the pharmacological effects of alcohol on behaviour. This *expectancy* effect is not limited to shock-giving since a similar phenomenon is apparent in the sexual response of male undergraduates to audiotapes depicting rape and sadistic aggression.[86]

There is a commonly held belief that alcohol increases the likelihood of an individual engaging in risk-taking behaviour.[87,88] This might obviously influence statistics on violent accidents, and indeed, some authors suggest that prior consumption of alcohol causes some subjects to commit acts of self-injury because it augments the tendency to incur greater than normal risks.[89] This phenomenon may also be important in relation to other acts of violence as some individuals tend to be more impetuous when drinking, and are thus more likely to be involved in violent crime.[27]

One neglected field of study is the potential interaction between alcohol and other drugs. For example, it is well known that alcohol in combination with hypnotic drugs, produces a greater degree of intoxication which may contribute to traffic accidents.[90] It is also likely that potentiation of the effects of barbiturates increases the probability of suicide attempts proving fatal. This type of action may also be important in other types of violence. For example, Paul[91] describes two disturbing cases where individuals consumed small doses of alcohol (equivalent to 1.2 pints (0.57-1.1 l) of beer) in conjunction with 1-2 tablets of Mandrax (a commercial hypnotic consisting of a mixture of methaqualone and diphenhydramine). In one case the mixture was taken inadvertently, whereas in the other it was taken intentionally to induce intoxication more rapidly and cheaply. In both cases extreme violence was directed to the police and other individuals unlucky enough to become involved.

Because testosterone is important in many mammalian species for the expression of male aggressive behaviour,[92] some investigators have examined the possibility that alcohol influences this activity by changing circulating androgen levels.[72,93,94] The initial results have proved disappointing; which is perhaps unsurprising, as it is well known that alcohol can depress blood testosterone levels,[95,96,97] a change the reverse of the one needed to validate the hypothesis. Having said this, Mendelson and Mello[72] point out that most studies on man have involved the taking of single or infrequent blood samples for analysis. Factors such as circadian variation in hormone levels may confound the results. Unless repeated samples are taken and correlated temporally with observed behaviour, it is virtually impossible to conclude anything about the influence of alcohol on hormones and aggression. Nevertheless, Rada, Laws and Kellner[59] report that, although the plasma testosterone levels of rapists and child molesters were within the normal range, a group of very violent rapists had significantly higher titres than other rapists or normal individuals. It should be noted, however, that this sub-group was very small (N=5), which emphasises the urgent need for further studies.

Having considered the associations between alcohol ingestion and violence in general, it is convenient to examine the relationship between this drug and specific kinds of violence.

Petty Crime, Felony and Homicide. The motivations for this heterogeneous category of crimes are likely to be varied. It is inevitable that there will be some overlap between this category and others described in this chapter. Fatal incidents which are the result of quarrels between members of a family or violent sexual assault are obviously likely to be included in homicide statistics. Many of these crimes, however, do not involve interpersonal violence, and it is a moot point whether burglary, stealing and receiving stolen goods should be included in this discussion. One would be hard pressed to argue convincingly that an aggressive motivation is involved in many of these incidents. In some cases (e.g. robbery with violence), the primary motivation is presumedly personal gain, and violence is used as a means to that end. Another distinct type of crime involves interpersonal conflict which may escalate to assault. In such cases it is often difficult to establish responsibility since the victim may provoke the incident.[3,29] As mentioned earlier,[28] alcohol seems most involved with the latter type of incident where behaviour is impulsive rather than planned. In other crimes (e.g. robbery), drinking may actually be discouraged in order to avoid bungling of the crime through intoxication. There is also an association between petty crime and alcohol,[18,98,99] but it is probable that this relationship primarily involves the chronic aspects of alcoholism rather than the acute pharmacological effects of the drug.

Sexual Assault. Simple views on cause and effect in sexually related crime should be disregarded. One must initially investigate the epidemiology of rape and the psychology of the rapist, before attempting to implicate alcohol. The stereotype of the 'typical' rapist appears to be a myth, as case reports indicate a wide range of motivations and activities that receive the label of rape.[39] Some rapes appear to be carefully planned whereas others are clearly opportunistic. Rapists may be familiar to their victims or complete strangers;[100] they may or may not have a history of voyeurism, fetishism and exhibitionism,[40] can be hopelessly inadequate in their sexual relationships with women, or can be apparently happily married.[40]

Groth, Burgess and Holmstrom[101] identified three components of rape motivation which were 'power', 'anger' and 'sexuality'. Most authorities currently recognise that sexual and aggressive tendencies may be present to different degrees in particular cases.[59] Some sexual offenders use violence as a means to obtain sexual intercourse, while others require a degree of resistance to violence from the victim to achieve some form of sexual release.[40,102] Because of the evidence of diversity between rapists and rape situations, it seems quite possible that alcohol precipitates one kind of rape, has no effect on another, and even inhibits a third. Where the primary aim is sexual intercourse, the inhibiting effect of larger doses of alcohol on erection seem likely to prevent rape from taking place, although smaller doses could increase motivation and impulsiveness. In other cases where violence *per se* is a more significant feature, alcohol might increase the likelihood of assault.[8,39]

Violence Within the Family. It has already been pointed out that women from violent backgrounds are likely to choose husbands knowing that they also have a propensity for violence. It is quite possible that alcohol (through its pharmacological effects) acts directly to promote violence, but Hanks and Rosenbaum[5] have shown that this drug may also have an immediate but indirect effect. Women in this situation may unwittingly interact with men to 'ignite' the violence, especially when expressing (often reasonable) disapproval of their husband's drinking and drunken behaviour.

Suicide. Plausible explanations for raised BACs in individuals who attempt suicide, include the suggestion that drink provides 'Dutch Courage'[103] encouraging individuals to be impulsive. Drinking may change mood, and (as noted earlier) the direction of this change may vary according to personality. Some workers suggest that alcoholics are suicidal because they are depressed or depression-prone,[104] whereas others maintain that a state of 'hopelessness' is the key to suicidal intent in alcoholics and non-alcoholics.[105] Drinking may enhance these feelings. This suggestion is supported by a study by James,[11] who found that the great majority of successful suicides had been carried out some hours after drinking when euphoric feelings are likely to be replaced by dysphoria. Alcohol may also influence the suicide statistics via its interaction with other drugs, making a successful suicide more probable.

Accidental Injury. The role of alcohol in the causation of accidents also appears to vary with the type of incident considered.

Mackie[106] maintains that exercise before drinking can result in hypoglycaemia, with resulting weakness and an inability to maintain body temperature. This may be significant in cases of 'death-by-drowning'. On the other hand, gross intoxication may impair coordination and result in injury due to falling.[15]

The causation of driving accidents seems most complex. Moderate drinking may simply impair psychomotor performance increasing driver error. Selzer and Payne[13] also suggest that subconscious self-destructive urges (sometimes abetted by alcohol intoxication) are a major factor in the causation of some road accidents. However, there seem to be clear differences between the personalities of fatally injured male drivers (assessed in retrospect) and male suicides.[107] A detailed study revealed that only a tiny minority of traffic accidents could reasonably be deemed to have been suicide attempts.[108] Alcohol-induced willingness to take risks may be an important factor in such cases.

The Relationship Between Alcoholism and Violence

The statistical link between alcoholism and violence is usually interpreted in a number of ways. Alcoholism may be regarded as predisposing individuals towards violence. Alternatively, it may be held responsible for changes in the individual's social and environmental circumstances which increase the probability of being involved in some violent incident. Indeed, it may be maintained that there is no direct link between alcoholism and aggression, but that these two aspects of human behaviour are associated because they have a common cause. A variety of (not necessarily mutually exclusive) possibilities are discussed below.

Alcoholism as a Predisposer for Violence. This condition can predispose individuals towards violence in a number of ways. Since alcoholics drink more frequently than the general population, there is a greater likelihood that they will become involved in violence due to the acute pharmacological effects of alcohol. Another possibility is that chronic alcohol abuse leads to organic brain damage or some kind of psychiatric illness that is associated with violent behaviour. Ron[109] found gross morphological changes in the brain as a result of chronic alcohol abuse with evidence of associated psychological problems. Little effort seems to have been directed to examining the possibility that this contributes to violent behaviour. Similarly, few studies have investigated the role of 'alcoholic psychoses' in violence although it has been mentioned that morbid 'alcoholic jealousy' or 'threatening auditory hallucinations' may be involved in a few cases.[56]

Alcoholism as a Social Disadvantage. Alcoholism may also disrupt normal social relationships, reduce the ability to hold down a job, and produce a tendency to associate with other alcoholics. Lack of funds may predispose some individuals to use violence to obtain supplies of alcohol and food or to avoid capture. A worsening financial situation following the loss of a job or because the alcoholic spends too much money on alcohol may increase friction within the family, leading to violence.[6] In some cases rape may be precipitated by the social disruption which is secondary to chronic alcoholism.

Alcoholism and Violence as Linked by a Common Cause. Coid[56] (see also Chapter 6) concludes that there is a strong association between violence by alcoholics and a prior abnormality of personality. Such an antisocial personality may result from experiences of the effects of violence within the family. There is also some evidence suggesting a common genetic predisposition to alcohol abuse[110,111] and criminality.[112] Bohman[113] concludes, however, that whilst there is evidence for a genetic predisposition for alcoholism, the situation as regards criminality is more ambiguous.

Implications for the Control of Alcohol-related Violence

Prevention

The prevention of alcohol-related violence clearly lies to a degree within the realms of political decision-making. Prohibition does not seem a practical solution to the problem, but the price of alcohol could be increased in real terms. This, it is argued, should reduce the *per capita* consumption of alcohol, perhaps decreasing the incidence of alcohol-related problems. It could, however, be maintained that any such policy is socially unjust because lower income groups would be prevented from enjoying a traditional popular pastime, whilst politicians and the medical profession (who would generate the decision) would be amongst those least likely to be affected by higher prices. Certainly, such measures would not be popular amongst the majority of the electorate.

Another possibility is to add some drug to alcoholic beverages to counter the undesirable effects of alcohol. This seems unlikely in practice because (as noted earlier) alcohol may influence violence in a number of ways. Indeed, the suggestion that one has been drinking may be more important than alcohol *per se* in certain situations. Furthermore, the influence of alcohol on behaviour appears to depend on the social context or the individual's personality. Consequently, an added drug is unlikely to be any more specific for aggression than alcohol and might attenuate properties regarded as desirable in a majority of cases. Not only is it likely that the general public would oppose such measures, there is no known substance which presents itself as an obvious candidate for such a role.

Several useful things may still be done. In any programme designed to educate the public about the dangers of alcohol abuse, the association between alcohol and violence should be clarified. Alcohol could be made more difficult to obtain in situations where violence may be expected. Some Association Football matches are obvious candidates for such policies, but reducing the availability of alcohol will do nothing to influence the sociological determinants of 'football hooliganism'. The police should be educated about the true nature of alcohol-related violence because a great proportion of their work involves dealing with petty crime and minor outbreaks of public disorder in which alcohol may play a part.[19] The level of concern shown by the police differs from region to region in the UK.[37] Jeffs and Saunders[19] have shown that strict enforcement of licensing laws tends to reduce the number of arrests made in alcohol-related crime.

Treatment

Despite effective preventive measures, one must expect some casualties in societies where alcohol remains freely available. Studies show that alcoholism is strongly associated with recidivism,[98] but most men with drinking problems pass through prison without that fact being recorded.[99] A combination of sociopathy and alcoholism carries a poor prognosis,[114] and many drinkers are re-convicted within 9 to 12 months of leaving prison.[99]

It is quite clear that any programme involving rehabilitation should take alcoholism into account,[99,115] and should be extended beyond the prison environment. Otherwise, individuals inevitably succumb to the same environmental, social and psychological pressures which led to their initial conviction. The outcome of different treatment strategies should be continuously monitored so that they can be adjusted for maximal effectiveness. Policies which may have a considerable effect on recidivism seem possible, but these are often viewed as expensive. However, when the costs are compared to those inevitably incurred in keeping individuals in prison, after providing the associated policework and legal proceedings, they are revealed as relatively cost-effective as well as socially desirable measures.

References

1. Shupe, L.M. 'Alcohol and crime. A study of the urine alcohol concentration found in 882 persons arrested during or immediately after commission of a felony', *Journal of Criminal Law and Criminology*, 1954, *44*, 661-4.

2. Nicol, A.R., Gunn, J.C., Gristwood, J., Foggit, R.H. and Watson, S.P. 'The relationship of alcoholism to violent behaviour resulting in long-term imprisonment', *British Journal of Psychiatry*, 1973, *123*, 47-51.

3. Virkkunen, M. 'Alcohol as a factor precipitating aggression and conflict behaviour leading to homicide', *British Journal of Addiction*, 1974, *69*, 149-54.

4. Goodwin, D.W. 'Alcohol in suicide and homicide', *Quarterly Journal of Studies on Alcohol*, 1973, *34*, 144-56.

5. Hanks, S.E. and Rosenbaum, C.D. 'Battered women: a study of women who live with violent alcohol-abusing men', *American Journal of Orthopsychiatry*, 1977, *47*, 291-306.

6. Byles, J.A. 'Violence, alcohol problems and other problems in disintegrating families', *Journal of Studies on Alcohol*, 1978, *39*, 551-3.

7. Rada, R.T. 'Alcoholism and forcible rape', *American Journal of Psychiatry*, 1975, *132*, 444-6.

8. Johnson, S.D., Gibson, L. and Linden, R. 'Alcohol and rape in Winnipeg', *Journal of Studies on Alcohol*, 1978, *39*, 1887-98.

9. Rada, R.T. 'Alcoholism and the child molester', *Annals of the New York Academy of Science*, 1976, *273*, 492-6.

10. Frankel, B.G., Ferrence, R.G., Johnson, F.G. and Whitehead, P.G. 'Drinking and self-injury; towards untangling the dynamics', *British Journal of Addiction*, 1976, *71*, 299-306.

11. James, I.P. 'Blood alcohol levels following successful suicide', *Quarterly Journal of Studies on Alcohol*, 1966, *27*, 23-9.

12. Haberman, P.W. and Baden, M.M. 'Alcoholism and violent death', *Quarterly Journal of Studies on Alcohol*, 1974, *35*, 221-31.

13. Selzer, M.L. and Payne, C.E. 'Automobile accidents, suicide and alcoholism', *Proceedings of the 3rd International Conference on Alcohol and Road Traffic* (ed. Havard, J.D.J.) London, 1962, 104-7.

14. Oppenheim, W.L. 'The "battered alcoholic syndrome"', *Journal of Trauma*, 1977, *17*, 850-6.

15. Evans, C.M. 'Alcohol, violence and aggression', *British Journal on Alcohol and Alcoholism*, 1980, *15*, 104-17.

16. Evans, C.M. 'Alcohol and sexual assault', *British Journal of Sexual Medicine*, 1982, *9*, 40-2.

17. Crawford, A., Hinton, J.W., Docherty, C.J., Dishman, D.J. and Mulligan, P.E. 'Alcohol and crime I. Self-reported alcohol consumption of Scottish prisoners', *Journal of Studies on Alcohol*, 1982, *43*, 610-13.

18. Horverak, O. 'The 1978 strike at the Norwegian Wine and Spirits Monopoly', *British Journal of Addiction*, 1983, *78*, 51-66.

19. Jeffs, B.W. and Saunders, W.M. 'Minimizing alcohol-related offences by enforcement of the existing licencing legislation', *British Journal of Addiction*, 1983, *78*, 67-77.

20. Heather, N. 'Relationships between delinquency and drunkenness among Scottish young offenders', *British Journal on Alcohol and Alcoholism*, 1981, *16*, 150-61.

21. Wolfgang, M.E. *Patterns in Criminal Homicide*, Philadelphia: University of Pennsylvania Press, 1958.

22. Tinklenberg, J.R. 'Alcohol and violence', in *Alcoholism: Progress in Research and Treatment* (eds Bourne, P. and Fox, R.), New York: Academic Press, 1973, pp. 195-210.

23. Parker, N. 'Murderers: A personal series', *Medical Journal of Australia*, 1979, *1*, 36-9.

24. Hart-Hanson, J.P. and Bjamason, O. 'Homicide in Iceland 1946-1970', *Forensic Science*, 1974, *4*, 107-17.

25. Gillies, H. 'Homicide in the West of Scotland', *British Journal of Psychiatry*, 1976, *128*, 105-27.

26. Lester, D. and Lester, G. *Crime of Passion: Murder and the Murderer*, Chicago: Nelson-Hall, 1975.

27. Lester, D. 'Temporal variation in suicide and homicide', *American Journal of Epidemiology*, 1979, *109*, 517-20.

28. Myers, T. 'Alcohol and violent crime re-examined: self-reports from two sub-groups of Scottish male prisoners', *British Journal of Addiction*, 1982, *77*, 399-413.

29. Wolfgang, M.E. and Strohm, R.B. 'The relationship between alcohol and criminal homicide', *Quarterly Journal of Studies on Alcohol*, 1956, *17*, 411-25.

30. Guze, S.B., Tuason, V.B., Gatfield, P.D., Stewart, M.A. and Picken, B. 'Psychiatric illness and crime with particular reference to alcoholism; studies of 233 criminals', *Journal of Nervous and Mental Diseases*, 1962, *134*, 512-21.

31. Yarvis, R.M. 'Psychiatric pathology and social deviance in 25 incarcerated offenders', *Archives of General Psychiatry*, 1972, *26*, 79-84.

32. California, Department of Public Health, Division of Alcoholic Rehabilitation. *Alcoholism and California: Criminal Offenders and Drinking Involvement: a Preliminary Analysis* (Publication No. 3), Berkeley, 1960.

33. American Medical Association. *Manual on Alcoholism*, Chicago: American Medical Association, 1968 (revised 1973).

34. McGeorge, J. 'Alcohol and crime', *Medical Science and the Law*, 1963, *3*, 27-48.

35. Robinson, C., Patton, J. and Kerr, W. 'A psychiatric assessment of criminal offenders', *Medical Science and the Law*, 1965, *5*, 140-6.

36. Lester, D. 'Alcohol and suicide and homicide', *Journal of Studies on Alcohol*, 1980, *41*, 1220-3.

37. Plant, M.A. and Pirie, F. 'Self-reported alcohol consumption and alcohol-related problems: a study in four Scottish towns', *Social Psychiatry*, 1979, 65-73.

38. MacAndrew, C. and Edgerton, R.B. *Drunken Comportment: A Social Explanation*, London: Thomas Nelson, 1969.

39. Amir, M. *Patterns in Forcible Rape*, Chicago: University of Chicago Press, 1971.

40. Rada, R.T. *Clinical Aspects of the Rapist*, New York: Grune & Stratton, 1978.

41. Gayford, J.J. 'The aetiology of repeated serious physical assaults by husbands on wives (wife battering)', *Medical Science and the Law*, 1979, *19*, 19-24.

42. Gerson, L.W. 'Alcohol-related acts of violence: who was drinking and where the acts occurred', *Journal of Studies on Alcohol*, 1978, *39*, 1294-6.

43. Gayford, J.J. 'Battered wives', *Medical Science and the Law*, 1975, *15*, 237-45.

44. James, I.P., 'Derham, S.P. and Scott-Orr, D.N. 'Attempted suicide — a study of 100 cases referred to a general hospital', *Medical Journal of Australia*, 1963, *1*, 375-80.

45. Sclare, A.B. and Hamilton, C.M. 'Attempted suicide in Glagow', *British Journal of Psychiatry*, 1963, 609-15.

46. Smith, J.S. and Davison, K. 'Changes in the pattern of admissions for attempted suicide in Newcastle upon Tyne during the 1960s', *British Medical Journal*, 1971, *4*, 412-15.

47. Norvig, J. and Nielsen, B. 'A follow-up study of 221 alcohol addicts', *Quarterly Journal of Studies on Alcohol*, 1956, *17*, 663-5.

48. Ritson, E.B. 'Suicide amongst alcoholics', *British Journal of Medical Psychology*, 1968, *41*, 235-42.

49. Palola, E.G., Dorpat, T.L. and Larson, W.R. 'Alcoholism and suicidal behaviour' in *Society, Culture and Drinking Patterns* (eds Pittman, D.J. and Snyder, C.R.), New York: John Wiley & Sons, 1962.

50. Jansson, B. 'A catamnestic study of 476 attempted suicides with special regard to the prognosis for cases of automatism', *Acta Psychiatrica Scandinavica*, 1962, *38*, 183-98.

51. Stenback, A. and Blumenthal, M. 'Relationship of alcoholism, hypochondria and attempted suicide', *Acta Psychiatrica Scandinavica*, 1964, *40*, 133-40.

52. Pluekhahn, V.D. 'Alcohol and accidental submersion from watercraft and surrounds', *Medical Science and the Law*, 1977, *17*, 246-50.

53. Galbraith, S., Murray, W.R., Patel, A.R. and Knill-Jones, R. 'The relationship between alcohol and head injury and its effect on the conscious level', *British Journal of Surgery*, 1975, *62*, 128-30.

54. Lacefield, D.J., Roberts, P.A. and Blossom, C. *Agricultural Aviation versus other General Aviation: Toxicological Findings in Fatal Accidents.* Prepared for US Department of Transportation, Federal Aviation Adminisration. (Report No. FAA-AM-78-31. US Nat. Tech. Inform. Serv.).

55. Machata, G. 'Alkohol und Unfall', *Hefte Zeitshrift für Unfallheilk*, 1978, *130*, 179-82.

56. Coid, J. 'Alcoholism and violence', *Drug and Alcohol Dependence*, 1982, *9*, 111-23.

57. Dight, S.E. *Scottish Drinking Habits*, London: Office of Population, Censuses and Surveys, Social Survey Division, HMSO, 1976.

58. Saunders, W.M. and Kershaw, P.W. 'The prevalence of problem drinking and alcoholism in the West of Scotland', *British Journal of Psychiatry*, 1978, *133*, 493-9.

59. Rada, R.T., Laws, D.R. and Kellner, R. 'Plasma testosterone levels in the rapist', *Psychosomatic Medicine*, 1976, *38*, 257-68.

60. McCrady, B., Paolino, T.J. and Longabaugh, R. 'Correspondence between reports of problem drinkers and spouses on drinking behaviour and

impairment', *Journal of Studies on Alcohol*, 1978, *39*, 1252-7.
61. Sobell, L. and Sobell, M. 'Validity of self-reports in three populations of alcoholics', *Journal of Consulting and Clinical Psychology*, 1978, *46*, 901-7.
62. Sobell, L.C., Maisto, S.A., Sobell, M.B. and Cooper, A.M. 'Reliability of alcohol abusers' self-reports of drinking behaviour', *Behavior Research and Therapy*, 1979, *17*, 157-60.
63. Morse, S.J. 'Diminished Capacity: A moral and legal conundrum', *International Journal of Law and Psychiatry*, 1979, *2*, 271-98.
64. Fingarette, H. *Crime Prevention: Perception*, Canadian Council on Social Development, Spring, 1981, 27-32.
65. Roizen, J. and Schneberk, D. 'Alcohol and Crime' in *Alcohol, Casualties and Crime*, Berkley: Social Research Group, 1978.
66. Room, R. 'Alcohol in casualties and crime: the current state of research and future directions', paper presented to the 24th International Institute of the Prevention and Treatment of Alcoholism, Zurich, 25-30, June, 1978.
67. Merek, Z., Widacki, J. and Hanausek, T. 'Alcohol as a victimogenic factor of robberies', *Forensic Science*, 1974, *4*, 119-23.
68. Smith, A.M. 'The complainant's condition in rape cases', *Medical Science and the Law*, 1979, *19*, 25-8.
69. Clark, L. 'The treatment of rape and rape victims within the Canadian criminal justice system; failure facts and theory', paper presented at the Research on Women Conference, Halifax, Nova Scotia, 1976.
70. Baldwin, J. and McConville, M. 'Sentencing problems raised by guilty pleas: an analysis of negotiated pleas in the Birmingham Crown Court', *The Modern Law Review*, 1978, (September), 544-58.
71. Grayham, K., La Rocque, L., Yetman, R., Ross, T.J. and Guistra, E. 'Aggression and bar-room environments', *Journal of Studies on Alcohol*, 1980, *41*, 277-92.
72. Mendelson, J.H. and Mello, N.K. 'Alcohol, aggression and androgens', *Aggression. Proc. A.R.N.M.D.* (ed. Frazier, S.H.), Baltimore: Williams & Wilkins, 1974, 225-47.
73. Boyatzis, R.E. 'The predisposition towards alcohol-related interpersonal aggression in man', *Journal of Studies on Alcohol*, 1975, *36*, 1196-207.
74. Taylor, S.P., Gammon, C.B. and Capasso, D.R. 'Aggression as a function of the interaction of alcohol and threat', *Journal of Personality and Social Psychology*, 1976, *34*, 930-41.
75. Bennet, R.M., Buss, A.H. and Carpenter, J.A. 'Alcohol and human physical aggression', *Quarterly Journal of Studies on Alcohol*, 1969, *30*, 870-6.
76. Conger, J.J. 'The effects of alcohol on conflict behaviour in the albino rat', *Quarterly Journal of Studies on Alcohol*, 1951, *12*, 1-29.
77. Abraham, K. 'Notes on the psychoanalytical investigation and treatment of manic-depressive insanity and allied conditions', *Selected Papers on Psychoanalysis: 1911*, London: Hogarth Press, 1927.
78. Cochrane, N. 'The role of aggression in the psychogenesis of depressive illness', *British Journal of Medical Psychology*, 1975, *48*, 113-30.
79. Miller, N.E. and Barry, H. 'Motivational effects of drugs: methods which illustrate some general problems in psychopharmacology', *Psychopharmacologia*, 1960, *1*, 169-99.
80. Kahn, R., McClelland, D.C. and Kahn, M. 'The effects of male social drinking and fantasy', *Journal of Personality and Social Psychology*, 1965, *1*, 441-52.
81. Cappell, H. and Latane, B. 'Effects of alcohol and caffeine on the social and emotional behaviour of the rat', *Quarterly Journal of Studies on Alcohol*, 1969, 30A, 345-56.

82. Cappell, H. and Herman, C.P. 'Alcohol and tension reduction. A review', *Quarterly Journal of Studies on Alcohol*, 1972, 32A, 33-64.

83. Carpentier, J.A. and Armenti, N.P. 'Some behavioral effects of alcohol on man' in *The Biology of Alcoholism: Vol. II* (eds B. Kissen and H. Beglater), New York: Plenum, 1972.

84. Taylor, S.P. and Gammon, C.B. 'Effects of type and dose of alcohol on human physical aggression', *Journal of Personality and Social Psychology*, 1975, *32*, 169-75.

85. Lang, A.R., Goeckner, D.J., Adesso, V.J. and Marlett, G.A. 'Effects of alcohol on aggression in male social drinkers', *Journal of Abnormal Psychology*, 1975, *84*, 508-18.

86. Farkas, G.M. and Rosen, R.C. 'Effect of alcohol on elicited male sexual response', *Journal of Studies on Alcohol*, 1976, *37*, 265-72.

87. Cohen, J. *Chance, Skill and Luck*, London: Pelican, 1960.

88. Sjoberg, L. 'Alcohol and gambling', *Psychopharmacologia*, 1969, *14*, 284-98.

89. Stengle, E. *Suicide and Attempted Suicide*, London: Penguin, 1964.

90. Saario, I. and Linnolia, M. 'Effect of subacute treatment with hypnotics alone, or in combination with alcohol, on psychomotor skills related to driving', *Acta Pharmacologia et Toxicologica*, 1976, *38*, 382-92.

91. Paul, D.M. 'Drugs and aggression', *Medical Science and the Law*, 1975, *15*, 16-21.

92. Leshner, A.I. 'A model of hormones and agonistic behavior', *Physiology and Behavior*, 1975, *15*, 225-35.

93. Dotson, L.E., Robertson, L.S. and Tuchfield, B. 'Plasma alcohol, smoking, hormone concentrations and self-reported aggression: a study in a social drinking situation', *Journal of Studies on Alcohol*, 1975, *36*, 578-86.

94. Persky, H., Smith, K.D. and Basu, G.K. 'Relation of psychologic measures of aggression and hostility to testosterone production in man', *Psychosomatic Medicine*, 1971, *33*, 265-77.

95. Badre, F.M. and Bartke, A. 'Effect of ethyl alcohol on plasma testosterone level in mice', *Steroids*, 1974, *23*, 921-7.

96. Cicero, T.J. and Badger, T.M. 'Effect of ethyl alcohol on the hypothalamic-pituitary-gonadal axis in the male rat', *Journal of Pharmacology and Experimental Therapeutics*, 1977, *201*, 427-33.

97. Van Theil, D.H. and Lester, R. 'Alcoholism: its effect on hypothalamic pituitary gonadal function', *Gastroenterology*, 1976, *71*, 318-27.

98. Gibbons, T.C.N. and Silberman, M. 'Alcoholism among prisoners', *Psychological Medicine*, 1970, *1*, 73-8.

99. Edwards, G., Hensman, C. and Peto, J. 'Drinking problems amongst recidivist prisoners', *Psychological Medicine*, 1971, *1*, 388-99.

100. Schiff, A.F. 'Statistical trends in rape', *Journal of Forensic Science and Sociology*, 1979, *19*, 95-106.

101. Groth, A.N., Burgess, A.W. and Holmstrom, L.L. 'Rape: power, anger and sexuality', *American Journal of Psychiatry*, 1977, *134*, 1239-43.

102. Abel, G.G., Barlow, D.H. and Blanchard, E.B. 'The components of rapists' sexual and arousal', *Archives of General Psychiatry*, 1977, *34*, 895-903.

103. McCullough, J.W. and Phillip, A.F. *Suicidal Behaviour*, Oxford: Pergamon Press, 1972.

104. Woodruff, R.A., Guze, S.B., Clayton, P.S. and Carr, D. 'Alcoholism and depression', *Archives of General Psychiatry*, 1963, *9*, 324-35.

105. Beck, A.T., Weissman, D. and Kovacs, M. 'Alcoholism, hopelessness and suicidal behavior', *Journal of Studies on Alcohol*, 1976, 66-77.

106. Mackie, I. 'Alcohol and aquatic disasters', *Medical Journal of Australia*, 1978, *65*, 652-3.
107. Shaffer, J.W., Perlins, A. and Schmidt, C.W. 'Assessment in absentia; new directions in the psychological autopsy', *Johns Hopkins Medical Journal*, 1972, *130*, 308-16.
108. Schmidt, C.W., Shaffer, J.W., Zlotouritz, H.I. and Fisher, R.S. 'Suicide by vehicular crash'. *American Journal of Psychiatry*, 1977, *134*, 175-8.
109. Ron, M.A. 'Brain damage in chronic alcoholism: a neuropathological, neuroradiological and psychological review', *Psychological Medicine*, 1977, *7*, 103-12.
110. Goodwin, D.W., Schulsinger, L.F. and Hermansen, L. 'Alcohol problems in adoptees raised apart from alcoholic biological parents', *Archives of General Psychiatry*, 1973, *28*, 238-43.
111. Goodwin, D.W., Schulsinger, L.F. and Moller, N. 'Drinking problems in adopted and non-adopted sons of alcoholics', *Archives of General Psychiatry*, 1974, *31*, 164-9.
112. Hutchings, B. and Mednick, S. 'Registered criminality in the adoptive and biological parents of registered male criminal adoptees' in *Genetic Research in Psychiatry* (eds Fieve, R.R., Brill, H. and Rosenthal, D.), Baltimore: Johns Hopkins University Press, 1975.
113. Bohman, M. 'Some genetic aspects of alcoholism and criminality', *Archives of General Psychiatry*, 1978, *35*, 269-76.
114. Schuckitt, M.A. 'Alcoholism and sociopathy — diagnostic confusion', *Quarterly Journal of Studies on Alcohol*, 1973, *34*, 157-64.
115. Speiker, G. and Sarver, C.R. 'Alcohol and crime', *British Journal on Alcohol and Alcoholism*, 1978, 184-9.

6 ALCOHOL, RAPE AND SEXUAL ASSAULT

Jeremy Coid

It is perhaps unsurprising that little research has been carried out on the specific association between alcohol and sexual assaults on females. Complexities of the interaction between alcohol and other forms of aggression have already been outlined, and the additional dimension of sexuality will further multiply them. This chapter therefore reviews the literature, summarising the scanty data actually available, and indicates areas where further research is likely to be worthwhile. Detailed discussion of the theoretical issues in sexual assault and various models of alcohol's interactions with violent behaviour have been avoided, and readers are referred to Box[1] and Pernanen[2] respectively for detailed reviews. Studies to be examined are restricted to sexual assault on females by adult males, primarily the criminal offence of rape. However, as there are few studies in which variables of alcohol, sexual and violent behaviour are simultaneously examined, speculation on links with other examples will sometimes be inevitable.

Three main areas are covered in this chapter. First, the epidemiological and clinical studies of rape that include data on alcohol. Secondly, the relevant findings from the rapidly developing field of psychological experiments on human aggression are summarised. Finally, the overriding socio-cultural influences on drinking associated with sexual behaviour and male-to-female aggression in society will be examined.

Epidemiology

Both the lay press and the scientific literature frequently refer to a 'strong' influence of alcohol on crimes of violence, including rape, usually based on official sources of statistics. Table 6.1 summarises the major studies of rape over the last 30 years from which data on alcohol consumption by offender and/or victim can be extracted.[3 to 13] First impressions suggest their assumptions are correct, but with a wide range of 34-72 per cent of rapes in which the victim, offender or both, consumed alcohol shortly before the offence. However, these findings must be put in perspective as they are 'one-number' estimates[2] involving two variables (rape and alcohol consumption) that, in fact, may be unrelated, and ignore other variables that might be influencing the findings. Only Amir[6] gives data on the rape-rate in the populations from which the samples were drawn. This is a serious omission, as any comparisons between percentages in different studies are otherwise meaningless, as recently shown in studies of homicide by mentally abnormal offenders.[14] Furthermore, there is no information on overall levels or patterns of alcohol consumption within the general population. At the individual subject level, little information is given on the quantity of alcohol consumed, and readers are lucky to find crude gradations such as 'drunk' or 'mild intoxication'.

Clearly, there is little similarity between the methodology of these studies for the purposes of useful comparison, and samples from a State Hospital[8,9] and prison[4] are undoubtedly biased. Intoxication *per se* could well predispose certain subjects' crimes to be reported, detected, and the individuals apprehended, charged, and their alcoholism directed towards a hospital disposal. Although other authors have attempted to obtain more representative samples from court cohorts,[12] or consecutive cases from police files[5 to 7,10] it is uncertain to what extent drinking by the participants had influenced police decision-making on whether to prosecute. Factors relating to the crime itself will influence the charge, and Evans[15] (see also Chapter 5) has pointed out that the distinction between rape and a lesser charge is often slight. For example, penetration with an inanimate object instead of a penis, may be at least as traumatic, but results in a charge of indecent assault, with further reductions of charge sometimes brought about at a later stage by plea bargaining.

A large number of rapes are included within the 'Dark Figure of Crime'[16] in that they are unreported, therefore making a reliable estmate of alcohol's involvement particularly difficult. In addition, legislative changes such as the introduction of the Sexual Offences (Amendment) Act 1977, can result in increased convictions in the following years. The problem is further compounded by apparent changes in reporting with time. Chappell[17] points out that the National Victimisation Survey carried out in the USA in 1967 suggested a ratio of 3 to 4 actual rapes for each case reported to the police, whereas a survey in two American cities some years later

Table 6.1: Details of Major Studies in which the Role of Alcohol in Rape has been Examined

Author	Location	Sample	Method	Result
Shupe (1954)[3]	Columbus, Ohio	42 persons arrested for rape	Urine analysis	21 (50%) had alcohol in their urine
Gebhard *et al.* (1965)[4]	Institute for Sex Research, Bloomington, Indiana	192 adult males convicted of sexual contact accompanied by force or threat with females 16 yrs or over	Interview of prisoners in different penal institutions	39% drunk at time; 15% mild or moderate intoxication
Amir (1967, 1971)[5,6]	Philadelphia	646 rape victims, 1,292 offenders, 1958 and 1960	Police files search, consecutive cases	34% single offenders; 63% multiple; Alcohol present in victim, offender, or both
MacDonald (1971)[7]	Denver	200 rape victims 1968-9	Police files search, consecutive cases	9/22 (41%) victims of group-rape drinking
Rada (1975, 1978)[8,9]	Atascadero State Hospital, California	77 convicted rapists	Case autobiographies, non-random selection	50% offenders drinking 10 beers or more at the time
Johnson *et al.* (1978)[10]	Winnipeg	217 rapes or attempted rapes 'founded' by police	Police files search	72% cases alcohol in offender, victim or both
Groth and Birnbaum (1979)[11]	Massachusetts and Connecticut	'Over 500 offenders'	Information from victims, hospital referrals, maximum-security hospital inmates, 2 correctional institutions	50% using alcohol and/or drugs prior to assault
Giroux *et al.* (1980)[12]	Montreal	230 cases rape and attempted rape, Jan. 1975-May 1978	Court cohort. Consecutive cases	59.4% defendants and/or victims had consumed alcohol
Wright and West (1981)[13]	6 English counties	209 rapes, 88 attempts recorded as genuine over 5-yr period. Individual and group assaults	Police files search. Consecutive cases	'a third drinking heavily' 4 drinks or more; 10-15% lesser quantity

found a 2:1 ratio. Thus, changes in victim's reporting behaviour may well have made a contribution to the rise of rape-rates seen in most industrialised countries since the war.

Finally, the figures appearing in official statistics bear little relation to the numbers actually reported to the police once the various stages of the criminal process are passed through. For example, Dietz[18] observed from FBI reports for the USA in 1975 that 51 per cent of forcible rapes were 'cleared by arrest', 58 per cent of these arrested adults were prosecuted, and 42 per cent of those prosecuted were found guilty of forcible rape, with an additional 12 per cent being convicted of lesser offences. Only 16 per cent of the rapes actually reported led to a conviction, with 22 per cent of these convictions being for a lesser offence. It is no easier to make reliable estimations of alcohol's involvement in sexual assault in the UK. Box[1] makes a conservative estimate from victimisation surveys that there are approximately 5,000 rapes per year in England and Wales (roughly four times the number recorded in criminal statistics). Of the 25 per cent actually recorded by the police as rape incidents, 10 per cent are prosecuted, 7 per cent are found guilty, and 6 per cent are finally sent to prison.

Alcohol in the Rape Situation

Data on situational findings will also be modified by these processes. However, it is important to examine in some detail what is more accurately known about rape from self-report studies for comparison with those in Table 6.1. The largest survey was carried out in 26 US cities in 1974-5, representative samples being obtained by interview from approximately 10,000 households in each location.[19] Only slightly over half the women interviewed had reported incidents to the police, with those failing to report considering it a private or personal matter, believing that nothing could be done, or that there was lack of proof. Assaults by unknown offenders were higher than in most previous studies (82 per cent), although a further control investigation into the willingness of subjects to report to the interviewers themselves showed that this was less likely when the offender had been a relative. Assaults were highest for young women, with a readjusted annual US urban rate of 243 rapes per 100,000 females in the 16-19-year age range, and attempted rape highest for the 20-24-year age range at 488 per 100,000.

Black and other minority women, the lower-income groups, unmarried, divorced and separated subjects and those whose activities took them away from home (school, work, etc.) were most frequently victimised. The offenders were mostly 21 years or older, except when more than one offender was involved when both victim and offender tended to be younger. In all cities rape was highly intraracial, but somewhat less so when the victim was white. Incidents were more frequent in the evening and at night, and in open public areas such as streets or parks. Most offences were committed by one person and involved one victim, and theft was an element in only a small number. Weapons were used in less than half the incidents, but appeared an effective means of intimidation in that proportionately more attacks became a completed rape when the offender was armed. Knives were the most common weapons. Seventy per cent of victims did something to protect themselves, and attempts at self-defence lessened the chances that the rape would be completed, but increased the chances of receiving additional injuries. Rapes by non-strangers (18 per cent) were more highly intraracial, mainly occurring in the participant's own home, with a single attacker more likely to be involved. The victims attempted to protect themselves as often as they called for help, and there was no difference in the proportion injured. Following these two strategies, however, callers less frequently needed hospital attention.

Unfortunately, the survey contains no information on alcohol, but perhaps the most important observation when comparing other studies is the lack of major differences in the rape situation when alcohol is present in the participants. Amir[5,6] has carried out the most extensive statistical analysis of variables related to alcohol, but has concluded that an overall association was not supported, as it was absent in two-thirds of all his cases. His results do show certain contrasts between situations where alcohol was present and when it was not, but ultimately give little impression of how it might influence the event itself.

The only major contrast was that alcohol was significantly associated with white victims and offenders, except in the case of black victims who had been drinking before the offence. This was interesting as the rape-rate by black offenders was 12 times that for whites in Philadelphia. Amir does not give an adequate explanation for this, and the main conclusion was that among the various combinations of drinking patterns, alcohol in the victim alone and in both victim and offender have stronger implications of causal relationship than other patterns, but without relating this to racial findings. Alcohol was found to be strongly associated with violence used by the offender, which was confirmed in Winnipeg.[10] In addition, Amir found that black offenders who had been drinking tended to commit violent rapes.

Alcohol was also significantly associated with sexual humiliation of a victim who had been drinking, primarily in the form of enforced fellatio, usually demanded by a black offender. Interestingly, non-drinking whites were more violent towards their victims than were non-drinking blacks, suggesting that drinking patterns could have contrasted between the racial sub-groups as well as attitudes towards women when drinking. The data allow little further in the way of speculation, and could well have been distorted by higher rates of criminalisation of blacks due to police decisions to prosecute (see Dietz[18]). Although numbers were small and the sample probably biased, it could be relevant that the only self-report study of rapists in the literature found no more than the expected percentage of blacks.[20]

Amir also found a significant association between planning by the offender and alcohol, particularly when alcohol was present in the victim alone. He believed that this supported the notion that it is easier to conquer a drinking female. However, as a large proportion of these victims were black, it could also suggest that the black rapists perceived drinking women as 'fair game'. Johnson, Gibson and Lindon[10] contrasted by finding that alcohol was more strongly associated with unplanned rapes in Winnipeg. The reason for this difference is unclear, but it is probably due to variation in what the authors themselves considered constituted a planned assault rather than major differences in drinking patterns between the two cities. The Winnipeg study[10] also suggested that drinking offenders tended to rape more 'vulnerable' females. These included intoxicated women, but the very old and the young, physically and mentally handicapped subjects and women vulnerable due to their situation (such as working late, living alone, or sleeping at the time of the assault) were also at risk. Time of offence showed a significant association with drinking on Fridays, Saturdays and Sundays in Philadelphia.[5,6] However, if the author's tables are re-examined, the incidents *not* involving alcohol also clustered at weekends (25 per cent on Saturday alone) suggesting that an increase in social interaction (which may or may not involve drinking) is more important than alcohol *per se*.

The most controversial of Amir's findings involved the concept of 'victim-precipitation', which was frequently linked with alcohol consumption by the victim. In such situations the victim is thought to agree to sexual relations but retracts before the actual act, or is not felt to react strongly enough when the suggestion is made by the subsequent offender. In many cases, Amir found that the woman had been drinking with the offender prior to being raped, usually in one of their homes. In recent years this concept has received strong criticism from feminist authors, primarily as it inappropriately shifts the blame for rape onto the victim (see Box[1]).

Drinking by Multiple Offenders

Wright and West[13] carried out a useful comparison of group attacks and offences involving solitary offenders in the UK. Multiple offenders tended to be under 21 years, included more non-whites, had a smaller proportion with a previous sexual offence and who had never had a previous history of psychiatric treatment. Victims were more likely to have been drinking beforehand and to sustain minor injuries (this contrasts with US studies where these victims sustain more extensive injuries). When violence occurred in individual attacks it was usually a response to escalating victim resistance, but violence in group attacks was almost invariably gratuitous. The context from which the attacks typically developed was very different, with group assailants carrying out the assault in a relatively light-hearted manner, seemingly without appreciation of their own responsibility in the group's actions. The authors concluded that whereas some assaults by individual offenders may reflect personal propensities or pathology, group rapes originate in the dynamics of youthful gangs. Groth and Birnbaum[11] elaborated on these dynamics, describing the experience of rapport, fellowship, and co-operation amongst group members, each of whom behave as they perceive the others expect them, validating themselves as group members in the process, occasionally competing, but also showing motives of anger and desire for power over the victim, as with single offenders. In most cases, one offender subsequently emerges as the originator of the assault, usually taking the initiative and being the first to sexually assault the victim. His co-defendants often provided additional courage and aided in holding her down.

Presence of alcohol in the group members seems another component influencing the group's dynamics. Indeed, the factors of rapport, friendship, validation as a group member, minor competition and conforming to group norms, may be as relevant to the ritual and process of a male group's drinking together as to raping together. Unfortunately, statistical analyses of group offences yield little useful information on the nature of alcohol's involvement or the rape itself. Amir believed the association was stronger than in single offences, finding alcohol involved in 63 per cent of incidents and with a higher frequency in the victims of these assaults. However, his analysis tends to obscure the wide range of situations possible, rather than providing a useful framework for further research.

MacDonald described four patterns in Denver[7] which he claimed were fairly typical. Firstly, a single girl walking home at night attacked by a group of intoxicated strangers, secondly, youths calling at a girl's house claiming to be relatives take advantage of the absence of other family members (no specific alcohol involvement). Thirdly, a woman is seized by several men after leaving a bar where she has been drinking. Fourthly, a frequent pattern which is seen in groups of Spanish-American youths involves picking up a group of girls, giving them drink or drugs, and taking them to a secluded spot to rape them. These descriptive observations tell us considerably more about alcohol's involvement than Amir's statistical analysis. In the first example, the dynamics of the group may be the primary factor in the decision to rape. In the third, the woman's drinking may both determine her selection as victim, and alter the men's attitude towards her during the assault leading to excessive violence. It might subsequently influence whether the offence is 'founded' by the police, especially if she had been drinking with her assailants, which often increases their chances of acquittal. In the last example, alcohol appears deliberately used as a means of overcoming the victim's resistance. Each of these patterns provide testable hypotheses for future research, and in preliminary studies could be crudely converted into variables for comparison in different situations of multiple rape.

The Alcoholic Rapist

Two studies have looked specifically at alcoholic rapists using reasonably reliable criteria for diagnosis. Rada[8,9] found that over a third of his series committed to a State Hospital were self-confessed alcoholics or had rigorous criteria for alcoholism in their case histories (alcoholism could have caused them to be sent to a State Hospital). Unsurprisingly, virtually all were drinking prior to the offence compared to one-fifth of the non-alcoholics. They were also slightly older and had less education than non-alcoholics, but Rada emphasised that they were not 'skid-row' types. He believed these alcoholics inflated the overall findings for those offenders who were drinking prior to the offence — an important factor not controlled in other studies. Rada concluded that in these offenders, rape was just one of a series of maladaptive and self-destructive behaviours resulting from the overall personality deterioration consequent upon the addiction.

Barnard, Holzer and Vera[21] carried out a more detailed comparison of 22 alcoholic and 60 non-alcoholic rapists seen prior to court appearance, using Rada's criteria but giving no data as to their selection. Alcoholics were significantly older, tended to be white, and all but one had been drinking on the day of the offence. Their drinking started before they left school, and formal education ended at a relatively early age. More had been rejected or dishonourably discharged from the army, and all had previous arrests with more previous convictions for sexual offences. There were also significantly more non-sexual violent offences in the criminal histories of the alcoholic group. A third chose relatives as victims, all but two of whom were natural or step-daughters. Both groups showed long-standing and multi-faceted histories of disturbed behaviour, but alcoholics were the more severely disturbed in the amount and pattern of deviant behaviour which appeared earlier in their life histories. These tend to weaken Rada's assumption that alcohol dependence is the crucial factor in these alcoholics' rape behaviour. Rather, they support the conclusion of a recent literature review on alcoholism and violent behaviour[22] that offenders tend to comprise a sub-group of alcoholics with severe underlying personality disorders, predisposing them both to repetitively violent behaviour of various forms and their alcoholism.

Experimental Studies of Sexual and Aggressive Behaviour

Despite traditional assumptions that alcohol influences both aggressive and sexual behaviour, it was not until the early 1970s that research programmes began to systematically investigate these areas. Progress has now been made to the extent of challenging the traditional disinhibition model as too simplistic. The modifications emphasise alcohol's alteration of perception in the individual, the attribution of a threat to certain situations, and the expectancy of the subject when alcohol has been consumed (see refs 23 and 24). This section will provide an update on those studies relevant to alcohol and sexual assault.

Alcohol and Human Sexual Response

Kaplan[25] described the human sexual response as a highly rational and orderly sequence of physiological events, the object of which is to prepare the bodies of the mates for reproductive union. However, necessary sexual stimulation is profoundly influenced by personal experiences, cultural expectations, and the immediate situation in which the sexual act takes place. A further problem is the degree to which sexual assault can be considered within the framework of research into ordinary sexual behaviour, as the only relevant factor is the influence of alcohol on the physiological response of obtaining an erection and ejaculation by the offender. Bearing in mind these limitations, research has consistently shown a significantly negative linear relationship between alcohol and physiological responsiveness in both male and female drinkers.[26 to 29] Farkas and Rosen[26] found that in response to an erotic film there was a slight, but statistically significant facilitation of the amplitude of penile tumescence at low blood-alcohol concentrations (BACs), but the rate and extent decreased with increasing BAC. Malatesta, Pollack, Wilbanks and Adams[30], examined the effect on male orgasmic-ejaculatory response by asking 24 males to masturbate to sexually explicit videotapes. Latency time for ejaculation correlated significantly with BAC. As BAC increased, sexual arousal, pleasurability and intensity of orgasm decreased, whereas the difficulty in obtaining orgasm increased.

In the crude mechanical terms of obtaining an erection and ejaculating, alcohol seems likely to depress the sexual response of the rapist. It is naïve to merely conclude that alcohol predisposes men not to rape, as this simplistic analysis has a wider importance in two areas. First, it may provide insight into certain situational factors, e.g. the association between humiliation of the victim and alcohol (p. 166), indeed Groth and Birnbaum[11] have described how certain offenders will demand fellatio when unable to obtain an erection. Secondly, it gives further support to the claim that rape and other forms of sexual assault are acts of aggression against women using the genitalia as weapons with little or no sexual gratification. This feminist perspective (see ref. 31) is further supported by psychodynamic explanations of rape.[11]

Expectancy

Wilson[32] has concluded in a detailed review that (i) subjects' *expectancies* of the effect of alcohol can have profound effects on sexual behaviour; (ii) the physiological effect and the subjects' expected effect are quite separate; and (iii) the latter can override the former. This would provide one reasonable mechanism enabling intoxicated males to successfully rape (or indeed penetrate in a non-violent context) when the physiological influences are in the opposite direction. Two methodological approaches have been employed to measure expectancy effects: the subjects can be persuaded by the experimenter that the consumed alcohol will have a particular effect on their sexual arousal, or alternatively they are informed that they have consumed alcohol and their own assumptions are left uninfluenced by the experimenter. Wilson and Lawson[27] showed significantly increased penile tumescence in male subjects who believed they had consumed tonic water in response to erotic stimuli, irrespective of actual alcohol content. Wilson[32] later concluded that the individual's personal belief system was the major determinant of the effect of alcohol on sexual arousal — at least at moderate levels of intoxication (this personal belief system will itself be modified by the society to which the individual belongs).

Lang, Searles, Lauerman and Adesso[33] suggested that drinking alcohol not only permitted more interest in taboo sexual stimuli, but enabled individuals to intensify their attention by attributing responsibility to the state of intoxication. By employing an instrument designed to measure their subjects' levels of sexual guilt, these authors found a group with high recorded levels who believed they had consumed alcohol, showed a linear increase in the time they viewed erotic slides as the content became more pornographic, irrespective of the actual beverage content they had consumed. In contrast, their counterparts who believed they had consumed only non-alcohol beverages showed significantly shorter times. Males with moderate or low sex-guilt were not affected by beverage or expectancy, generally increasing viewing as content became more explicit, and indicating that individual characteristics, such as sexual guilt, are simultaneously involved in the expectation effect.

Individual Differences between Subjects

The expectation effect is particularly marked in studies of 'deviant' stimuli. Unfortunately, few studies have been carried out with drinking subjects in this area of research of major potential. Two studies[34,35] of non-drinking subjects have compared rapists and non-rapists when played audiotaped depictions of consenting sexual acts and rape. Whereas non-rapists showed higher arousal in both self-report and penile tumescence measures to consenting depictions, rapists showed approximately equal tumescence to both depictions. Abel and his colleagues[34] found that more violent rapists tended to be more sexually aroused by rape depictions than consenting sex. Importantly, individual differences in arousal to deviant stimuli are apparent within the general (non-institutionalised) population. Although more authors report relatively little sexual arousal to rape depictions in their subjects, Hinton, O'Neill and Webster[36] made the important observation that many do actually respond to deviant stimuli. Abel *et al.*[34,37] have developed a 'rape index' (a ratio of sexual arousal induced by rape portrayals to that following consenting sex portrayals), arguing that it serves as an objective index of the proclivity to rape, with certain men having an arousal to rape depictions greater or equal to consenting ones. Research by Malamuth[38] in a prison population suggested there are individuals with relatively strong inclinations to aggress against women. Quinsey, Chaplin and Carrigan[39] provided some support for the predictive validity of this measure, showing that it successfully predicted recidivism following discharge of sex offenders from a psychiatric institution. These findings lend support to the concept of there being a 'spectrum' of likelihood by males to assault females in the general population, with certain individuals having relatively strong inclinations that might be measurable using objective instruments. The influence of alcohol could be further examined using these developments.

Content of the Deviant Stimuli

Qualitative manipulation of the content of deviant stimuli presented to subjects has a major influence on results, a finding that correlates with observations of pornographic literature. Content analyses have revealed that a large amount of hard-core pornography[40] and an increasing amount of soft-core erotica[41] incorporate rape themes. This suggests that these may sexually arouse many consumers who are not actual rapists, but whose interests are clearly being met by the publishers. Once again the influence of alcohol through an expectancy effect was demonstrated by Briddell, Rimm, Caddy, Drawitz, Sholis and Wunderlin[42] measuring penile tumescence in normal subjects whilst playing tape recordings of erotic narratives describing mutually enjoyable heterosexual intercourse, forcible rape, and non-sadistic aggression. Subjects who believed they had consumed alcohol generally experienced a greater level of penile tumescence, but the expectancy effect was most marked for the forcible rape tape.

A major finding from this area is that the victim's reaction within the rape depiction has a crucial effect, with relatively little arousal by normal subjects when the victim is portrayed as abhoring the assault. In contrast, when the victim is portrayed as becoming involuntarily sexually aroused by what is happening to her (a typical depiction in pornography) sexual arousal in subjects is found to be as high or even non-significantly higher than arousal to consenting depictions.[43,44] More recently, Malamuth and Check[45] confirmed the added importance of individual personality differences between subjects. They found that the resulting sexual arousal to depictions, manipulated along dimensions of the woman's degree of consent and experience of pain, was not just an isolated response, but clearly associated with other measures of sexually aggressive tendencies in their subjects. By dividing them into two groups according to self-reported likelihood to rape, both groups were less aroused by the non-consenting depiction. However, when the depiction was manipulated to show the woman becoming sexually aroused, subjects with a higher self-reported likelihood to rape showed greater arousal to non-consenting than consenting scenes.

These findings illustrate the need to examine alcohol's effects on carefully separated groups of subjects according to personality and other individual differences. Developments in this area are particularly encouraging, but have still not clearly shown to what extent convicted rapists can be considered to have personality or other individual characteristics that are extreme examples of those present in the general population ('a spectrum' of severity model), or suffer from severe manifestations of psychopathology at the individual level (broadly conforming to an 'illness' model). A sample of convicted offenders is, however, unlikely to be heterogeneous, and these techniques may not shed much light on certain highly abnormal individuals. For example, Rada[9] made the interesting observation that in a small number of offenders in his sample, alcohol appeared to trigger certain physical sensations and sexual fantasies (often violent and bizarre), not present in the sober state. However, at the general level these techniques could shed further light by determining whether alcohol can overcome the negative effects on sexual arousal of disgust or pain depicted in the victim, a situation more relevant to actual rape. Further refinements might also examine the contribution of expectancy and individual differences and their interaction with alcohol.

Socio-cultural Influences

Wilson[32] has proposed a social-learning model for the influence of alcohol on sexual and aggressive behaviour. He proposed that as alcohol visibly impairs sensorimotor functions, this provides an ideal target of mis-attribution for violation of the normal code of conduct within society, facilitating the inference that social behaviour is similarly affected. The situations in which alcohol is consumed define sets of social role conditions that legitimise otherwise unacceptable actions. Here, the alcohol can be seen as a cue or discriminative stimulus for sexual behaviour, and the physiological changes perceived after consuming alcohol influence the cognitive labelling an individual gives to his situation. This correlates with the expectancy effect. The hypothesis does not explain what in turn, influences an individual's expectancy of how he will behave after drinking, or what he perceives as permissible whilst drinking by the society of which he is a member. Wilson acknowledged the importance of anthropological findings as a basis for his theories, particularly the work of MacAndrew and Edgerton.[46] In this final section, two separate socio-cultural approaches are taken to examine the influence of alcohol on sexual assault. First, the studies of 'drunken comportment' on sexual behaviour. Secondly, the attitudes towards sexuality and aggression within individual cultures, irrespective of drinking behaviour, and the extent to which drinking behaviour might be associated with these attitudes.

Anthropological Studies

Chapter 7 outlines the major findings of MacAndrew and Edgerton[46] that (i) certain societies fail to exhibit disinhibition after consuming alcohol; (ii) time and circumstances of drinking affect behaviour; (iii) drunken comportment is limited by social controls within these societies; (iv) drunken individuals show selectivity of targets for drunken aggression; (v) societies set aside 'Time Out' for drunken behaviour; and (vi) patterns of drunkenness change within individual societies over time. The same principles apply to sexual behaviour. For example, the Tarahumara Indians of Mexico provide 'Time Out' in the form of *fiestas* or *tesquinadas.* These people are highly reserved in everyday life, and their women are described as abnormally timid and puritanical, yet become 'quite free' when slightly intoxicated. At these times, when drinking plays a prominent role, a certain amount of licensed promiscuity and wife-exchange is evident. Intoxication itself was always blamed for such behaviour and was used as an excuse for a high proportion of transgressions that took place in Tarahumara society *coinciding* with these occasions. The example further demonstrates that Tarahumara women showed 'selectivity of object' for their sexual favours, as these did not extend to outsiders. Even though drunk, the women did not mix with strangers at fiestas, as those who were known to have had sexual relations with Mexicans were avoided for fear of disease.

The Zapotecs also sanction certain forms of deviant behaviour in intoxicated individuals.[47] Tolerance of sexual behaviour in their society was governed by shared norms. Although these extended to prohibit incest and adultery, such offences were often tolerated and actually relatively frequent. The only extra-marital sexual liaisons that were likely to be punished, occurred between socially distant individuals, and the only observed examples of sexual assault were public attempts to fondle the breasts of young girls. Both forms of deviancy were considered 'understandable' behaviour by the Zapotecs when the individual was intoxicated, otherwise they could only be perpetrated by an 'abnormal member' as Zapotec society provided ample opportunity for sexual relations.

Rape in Society

In a similar way Toner[48] has claimed that rape flourishes in societies that encourage it, and that the apparent strength of both male and female sex drive depends on the demands of individual cultures. This is supported by Sanday's[49] study of the incidence, meaning and function of rape in 156 primitive societies. Her sample was broadly divided into 'rape-prone' and 'rape-free' societies. Rape-prone are societies in which sexual assault of women is either culturally allowable or else largely overlooked, such as the Gusii of the Kenyan highlands whose rape-rate in 1955-6 was over three times that of the USA.[50] In these societies men are poised as a social group against women, and in some examples entry into the adult male or female group is marked by rituals involving rape, e.g. the Kikuyu of East Africa.[51] Sanday[49] described other examples where rape preserved the ceremonial integrity of the male group, signifying its status above women. Themes of women as 'property' are found in these societies where an aggrieved husband is financially compensated for the rape of his wife by another man, or when an adulterous woman is gang-raped by her husband and his unmarried compatriots.

Rape-free societies contrast with greater sexual equality and the shared idea that the two sexes are complementary or mutually indispensible. Most importantly, other forms of interpersonal violence are also uncommon in rape-free societies, leading Sanday to believe that men are not necessarily prone to rape, but when interpersonal violence is a way of life, the violence frequently has a sexual form of expression. Thus, it is not difficult to appreciate parallels with the way a society may shape its drunken aggression and this body of literature challenges the idea that a drunken assault is markedly different in motivation than an assault when sober. This viewpoint tends to place rape and other forms of sexual assault squarely within the overall patterns of violent behaviour common to each individual society. In each example, alcohol only assumes the degree of importance that the society attributes to it.

Industrialised Society

MacAndrew and Edgerton[46] believed that their findings applied equally to industrialised societies, but that these features were less apparent due to their plurality and heterogeneity. Sociological theories of deviancy have attempted to explain statistical associations between violent crime and membership of the lower social classes. This was observed by Amir in Philadelphia, who also confirmed that rapes tend to occur in socially deprived areas with the highest rates of other violent crime. He concluded that his subjects could be placed within the 'subculture of violence,' present among the lowest social classes and disenfranchised, where the prime value is the use of physical aggression as a demonstration of masculinity and toughness.[52] The importance of alcohol in sexual assault again depends on the extent to which it plays a part in the social interactions between sections of society where violence is frequent. Attitudes towards aggressive male sexuality at different levels of society may not be so different despite apparent contrasts in what is considered to be acceptable aggressive behaviour. Box[1] believes that many males from the higher social classes are equally coercive and exploitive, yet have greater access to females because of their status within society. This derives from differences in what is considered 'acceptable' as coercion and who is allowed to apply it. Studies of American college undergraduates also suggest that coercive sexuality may be a natural standard at all levels of Western society, a theory proposed by Clark.[53] A series of 291 women students[54] reported 1022 offensive incidents with their dates over a nine-month period, 20 per cent reported forcible attempts at intercourse accompanied by the threat of pain. No incidents were reported to the police. Similarly, 25 per cent of a series of undergraduate males[55] reported having made at least one attempt at coital access with a rejecting female, during the course of which physical coercion was utilised to the extent that the female objected. In a quarter of this sub-group, the male students were 'under the influence' of alcohol, but this theory suggests that they were already predisposed to behave aggressively.

Alcohol and the Criminal Process

Feminist authors have increasingly argued that attitudes towards coercive sexuality within Western society disadvantage women who have been sexually assaulted, tipping justice in favour of the offender. In England and Wales rape is sexual intercourse with a woman, not a wife, against her will by fear, force or fraud. Penetration can occur to any degree, and boys under 14 years are considered incapable of the offence. In court, it is necessary for the prosecution to convince the jury that penetration took place, the accused did it, the woman did not consent, and the man knew she did not consent. The most usual defence is to attempt to convince the jury that the woman consented or the man mistakenly thought she consented. Intoxication in either participant (particularly the woman) gives considerable scope to the defence. Furthermore, although a woman who is so intoxicated by alcohol or drugs is deemed incapable of consent, she is likely to have considerable difficulty in demonstrating that she did not consent or that she would not have consented when sober.

Drinking by women therefore appears to undermine their credibility as rape victims. LeGrand[56] examined the police decision-making process over whether to prosecute, and estimated that approximately 20 per cent of complaints are rejected as 'unfounded'. This is usually determined by the degree of consent expressed or thought to be implied by the demeanour of the victim, particularly if entering into a vulnerable situation (typically by becoming intoxicated with a strange man who has been buying her drinks all evening in a bar). Similar decision-making processes are seen amongst judges, and a study of their attitudes towards rape cases[57] revealed that they divided rapes into three types according to credibility: (i) 'genuine' victims — with no problem identifying the circumstances as forcible rape, mostly involving a brutal attack by a stranger on an unsuspecting victim; (ii) 'consensual intercourse' — where the judge felt the victim was 'asking for it', such as a pick-up in a bar; and (iii) 'female vindictiveness' — where the complainant was thought to be trying to 'get even' with a man, e.g. an ex-husband or boyfriend. The likelihood of eventual conviction may depend on the extent to which characteristics of the case approximate to stereotypes of rape held by the criminal justice personnel.[58] Black women, women who allegedly engaged in 'misconduct', women picked up in bars, women acquainted with the defendant, showing little physical injury, and failure to report the incident promptly, are all factors reducing the likelihood of coming to trial and of finally securing a conviction. Similar factors may account for Giroux, Boyer and Lamontagne[12] finding that acquittal in court in Montreal is significantly more common when the defendants had been drinking.

Conclusion

It is impossible to make a confident estimate of the extent to which alcohol consumption and sexual assault are associated from available studies. Indeed, merely observing incidences of drinking in victim and offender is unlikely to reveal useful information unless more sophisticated approaches are used. What is strikingly apparent from the statistical analyses of various studies is a *lack* of major contrasts between sexual assaults when alcohol is present and when it is absent. One exception was an apparent contrast between black and white offenders which remains unexplained, but may be due to differences in rape behaviour, attitudes towards women, and patterns of drinking within these sub-groups. This emphasises a need to re-examine these behavioural patterns with studies using more homogenous sub-groups. Particular attention should be paid to what consuming alcohol means to the individuals involved, rather than merely observing whether it is consumed or not.

Psychological research has attempted to fulfill these suggestions within laboratory settings and can complement clinical research. Although alcohol affects the rapist physiologically, making it more difficult to obtain an erection, his expectancy of subsequent behaviour may be of greater importance. One major question in this area of research is whether alcohol can facilitate rape by overcoming factors in the rapist that would normally make such behaviour less likely, particularly the perception of pain and distress in the victim. If this could be clearly demonstrated, further experiments might begin to examine whether such an effect was due to alterations in the rapist's perception of the victim or the situation, and the extent to which personality differences interacted with alcohol.

Individual differences between subjects and idiosyncratic reactions to alcohol have not been closely examined in this chapter, which has tended to examine overviews of the larger samples available. None of the clinical studies have attempted to sub-divide their subjects for comparison, whether examining the rapist himself or the rape. Clearly, neither are homogeneous. Gibbens and colleagues[59,60] have attempted to categorise rapists into three behavioural groups according to criminal histories; Bowden[61] has proposed a typology based on behaviour and psychiatric diagnosis; and Groth and Birnbaum[11] divided rape itself into three categories according to the dynamics and motivation for the offence. No current system is entirely satisfactory, although the last-mentioned is now the most widely accepted and may initially be used to crudely compare different patterns of rape and drinking behaviour.

A deliberate attempt has been made to lead the reader away

from simplistic examination of single variables in alcohol and sexual assault, and it is hoped these will be perceived as dependent on the socio-cultural influences or the situation in which they occur. Alcohol clearly has important symbolic and ritualistic significance in different societies, and may determine a variety of different factors such as choice of victim, the degree of injury and humiliation she may suffer, the likelihood she will report the assault, and the degree of culpability she herself may be perceived as having for the offence by other members of society. All these factors will ultimately influence research findings in this area.

There has been no intention of overstating the anthropological and sociological approach, but the pharmacological and physiological influences which are of major importance in the processes that prepare an individual for both sexual and aggressive behaviour have been documented in Chapters 2 and 3. In addition, this general overview has not taken into account the small proportion of highly abnormal individuals whose aggressive and sexual behaviour is neither governed by societies' norms nor easily explained by socio-cultural theories. They have not yet been measured within the context of experimental psychological research, but are encountered within clinical practice. Clearly, it is important to adhere to Pernanen's[2] recommendation that a multi-disciplinary approach be taken to future research into alcohol and criminal behaviour. This is especially relevant to the study of alcohol's influence on sexual assault.

Acknowledgement

I would like to thank Professor Griffith Edwards and Dr Paul Bowden for their advice on the manuscript.

References

1. Box, S. *Power, Crime and Mystification*, Tavistock Studies in Sociology, London: Tavistock Publications, 1983.
2. Pernanen, K. 'Theoretical aspects of the relationship between alcohol use and crime' in *Drinking and Crime* (ed. Collins, J.J.), London: Tavistock Publications, 1982.
3. Shupe, L.M. 'Alcohol and crime. A study of the urine alcohol concentration found in 882 persons arrested during or immediately after the

commission of a felony', *Journal of Criminal Law and Criminology*, 1954, *44*. 661-4.

4. Gebhard, P.H., Gagnon, H.H., Pomeroy, W.B. and Christenson, C.V. *Sex Offenders: An Analysis of Types*, New York: Harper & Row, 1965.

5. Amir, M. 'Alcohol and forcible rape', *British Journal of Addiction*, 1967, *62*, 219-32.

6. Amir, M. *Patterns in Forcible Rape*, Chicago, University of Chicago Press, 1971.

7. MacDonald, J.M. *Rape Offenders and their Victims*, Springfield, Illinois: Charles C. Thomas, 1971.

8. Rada, R.T. 'Alcoholism and forcible rape', *American Journal of Psychiatry*, 1975, *132*, 444-6.

9. Rada, R.T. *Clinical Aspects of the Rapist*, New York: Grune & Stratton, 1978.

10. Johnson, S.D., Gibson, L. and Linden, R. 'Alcohol and rape in Winnipeg 1966-1975', *Journal of Studies on Alcohol*', 1978, *39*, 1887-94.

11. Groth, A.M. and Birnbaum, H.J. *Men who Rape: the Psychology of the Offender*, New York: Plenum Press, 1979.

12. Giroux, J., Boyer, R. and Lamontagne, Y. 'Les causes de viol entendues dans le district judiciaire de Montreal entre 1975 et 1978: Une enquete retrospective', *Canadian Journal of Criminology*, 1980, *23*, 173-90.

13. Wright, R. and West, D.J. 'Rape: A comparison of group offences and lone assaults', *Medicine, Science and the Law*, 1981, *21*, 25-30.

14. Coid, J. 'The epidemiology of abnormal homicide and murder followed by suicide', *Psychological Medicine*, 1983, *13*, 855-60.

15. Evans, C.M. 'Alcohol and sexual assault', *British Journal of Sexual Medicine*, 1982, *9*, 40-2.

16. Wiles, P. 'Criminal statistics and sociological explanations of crime' in *The Sociology of Crime and Deviancy, Volume 1. The British Tradition*, (eds Carson, W.G. and Wiles, P.), Oxford: Martin Robertson, 1971.

17. Chappell, D. 'Forcible rape and the criminal justice system: Surveying present practises and projecting future trends' in *Sexual Assault* (eds Walker M.J. and Brodsky S.L), Lexington Books, 1976.

18. Dietz, P.E., 'Social factors in rapist behavior' in *Clinical Aspects of the Rapist*, (ed. Rada, R.T.), New York: Grune & Stratton, 1978.

19. McDermott, M.J. *Rape Victimization in 26 American Cities*, Albany, New York: Criminal Justice Research Center, 1979.

20. Smithyman, S.L. 'Characteristics of 'undetected' rapists' in *Perspectives on Victimology* (ed. Parsonage, W.H.), London: Sage, 1979.

21. Barnard, G.W., Holzer, C. and Vera, M. 'A comparison of alcoholics and non-alcoholics charged with rape', *Bulletin of the American Academy of Psychiatry and the Law*, 1979, *7*, 432-40.

22. Coid, J. 'Alcoholism and violence', *Drug and Alcohol Dependence*, 1982, *9*, 1-13.

23. Taylor, S.P. 'Alcohol and human physical aggression' in *Alcohol, Drug Abuse and Aggression*, (eds Gottheil E., Druley, K.A., Skoloda, T.E. and Waxman, H.M.), Springfield, Illinois: Charles C. Thomas, 1983.

24. Pihl, R.O. 'Alcohol and aggression: a psychological perspective' in *Alcohol, Drug Abuse and Aggression* (eds Gottheil, E., Druley, K.A., Skoloda, T.E. and Waxman, H.M.), Springfield, Illinois: Charles C. Thomas, 1983.

25. Kaplan, H.S. *The New Sex Therapy: Active Treatment of Sexual Dysfunction*, New York: Brunner/Mazel, 1974.

26. Farkas, G.M. and Rosen, R.L. 'Effect of alcohol on elicited male sexual response', *Quarterly Journal of Studies on Alcohol*, 1976, *37*, 265-72.

27. Wilson, G.T. and Lawson, D.M. 'Expectancies: alcohol and sexual arousal in male social drinkers', *Journal of Abnormal Psychology*, 1976, *85*, 587-94.
28. Wilson, G.T. and Lawson, D.M. 'The effects of alcohol on sexual arousal in women', *Journal of Abnormal Psychology*, 1976, *85*, 489-97.
29. Malatesta, V.J., Pollack, R.H., Crotty, T.D. and Peacock, L.J. 'Acute alcohol intoxication and female orgasmic response', *Journal of Sex Research*, 1982, *18*, 1-17.
30. Malatesta, V.J., Pollack, R.H., Wilbanks, W.A. and Adams, H.E. 'Alcohol effects on the orgasmic-ejaculatory response in human males', *Journal of Sexual Research*, 1979, *15*, 101-7.
31. Brownmiller, S. *Against Our Will: Men, Women and Rape*, London: Secker & Warburg, 1975.
32. Wilson, G.T. 'Alcohol and human sexual behaviour', *Behaviour Research and Therapy*, 1977, *15*, 239-52.
33. Lang, A.R., Searles, J., Lauerman, R. and Adesso, V. 'Expectancy, alcohol and sex guilt as determinants of interest in and reaction to sexual stimuli', *Journal of Abnormal Psychology*, 1980, *89*, 644-53.
34. Abel, G.G., Barlow, D.H., Blanchard, E.B. and Guild, D. 'The components of rapists' sexual arousal', *Archives of General Psychiatry*, 1977, *34*, 895-903.
35. Barbaree, H.E., Marshall, W.L. and Lanther, R.D. 'Deviant sexual arousal in rapists', *Behaviour Research and Therapy*, 1979, *17*, 215-22.
36. Hinton, J.W., O'Neill, M.T. and Webster, S. 'Psychophysiological assessment of sex offenders in a security hospital', *Archives of Sexual Behaviour*, 1980, *3*, 205-16.
37. Abel, G.G., Becker, J.V. and Skinner, L.J. 'Aggressive behavior and sex', *Psychiatric Clinics of North America*, 1980, *3*, 133-51.
38. Malamuth, N.M. 'Rape proclivity among males', *Journal of Social Issues*, 1981, *37*, 138-57.
39. Quinsey, V.C., Chaplin, T.C. and Carrigan, W.F. 'Biofeedback and signalled punishment in the modification of inappropriate sexual age preference', *Behaviour Therapy*, 1980, *11*, 567-76.
40. Smith, D.D. 'The social content of pornography', *Journal of Communication*, 1974, *26*, 16-33.
41. Malamuth, N.M. and Spinner, B.A. 'A longitudinal content analysis of sexual violence in the best-selling erotic magazines', *Journal of Sex Research*, 1980, *16*, 226-37.
42. Briddell, D.W., Rimm, D.C., Caddy, G.R., Drawitz, G., Sholis, D. and Wunderlin, R.J., 'Effects of alcohol and cognitive set on sexual arousal to deviant stimuli', *Journal of Abnormal Psychology*, 1978, *87*, 418-30.
43. Malamuth, N.M. and Check, J.V. 'Penile tumescence and perceptual responses to rape as a function of victim's perceived reactions', *Journal of Applied Social Psychology*, 1980, *10*, 528-47.
44. Malamuth, N.M. and Check, J.V.P. 'Sexual arousal to rape and consenting depictions: the importance of the woman's arousal', *Journal of Abnormal Psychology*, 1980, *89*, 763-6.
45. Malamuth, N.M. and Check, J.V.P. 'Sexual arousal to rape depictions: individual differences', *Journal of Abnormal Psychology*, 1983, *92*, 55-67.
46. MacAndrew, C. and Edgerton, R.B. *Drunken Comportment*: A Social Explanation, London: Thomas Nelson & Sons Ltd, 1969.
47. Selby, H.A. *Zapotec Deviance: The Covergence of Folk and Modern Sociology*, Austin: University of Texas Press, 1974.
48. Toner, B. *The Facts of Rape*, London: Arrow Books Ltd, 1982.
49. Sanday, P.R. 'The socio-cultural context of rape: A cross-cultural study',

Journal of Social Issues, 1981, *37*, 5-27.

50. Levine, R.A. 'Guisii sex offences: A study in social control' in *Sexual Behaviour in Canada: Patterns and Problems* (ed. Schlesinger B.), Toronto: University of Toronto Press, 1977.

51. Lambert, H.E. *Kikuyu Social and Political Institutions*, London: Oxford University Press, 1956.

52. Wolfgang, M.E. and Ferracuti, F. *The Subculture of Violence*, London: Tavistock, 1967.

53. Clark, L.M.G. 'Rape in Toronto: psychosocial perspectives in the offender' in *Sexual Behaviour in Canada: Patterns and Problems*, (ed. Schlesinger, B.) Toronto: University of Toronto Press, 1977.

54. Kirkpatrick, L. and Kanin, E. 'Male sex aggression on a university campus', *American Sociological Review*, 1957, *22*, 52-8.

55. Kanin, E. 'Male aggression in mating-courtship relationships', *American Journal of Sociology*, 1957, *62*, 197-204.

56. LeGrand, C. 'Rape and rape laws: sexism in society and law' in *Forcible Rape: The Crime, The Victim and The Offender* (eds Chappell, D., Geis, R. and Geis, G.), New York: Columbia University Press, 1977.

57. Bohmer, C. 'Judicial attitudes toward rape victims', *Judicature*, 1974, *57*, 303-7.

58. LaFree, G.D. Variables affecting guilty pleas and convictions in rape cases: toward a social theory of rape processing', *Social Forces*, 1980, *58*, 833-50.

59. Gibbens, T.C.N., Way, C. and Soothill, K.L. Behavioural types of rape', *British Journal of Psychiatry*, 1977, *130*, 32-42.

60. Soothill, K.L., Jack, A. and Gibbens, T.C.N. 'Rape: A 22-year cohort study', *Medicine, Science and the Law*, 1976, *16*, 62-9.

61. Bowden, P. 'Rape', *British Journal of Hospital Medicine*, 1978, *20*, 286-90.

7 SOCIO-CULTURAL FACTORS IN ALCOHOL-RELATED AGGRESSION

Jeremy Coid

Socio-cultural theories of disinhibition have become increasingly important to the study of alcohol-related aggression in recent years, as the prominence given to biological studies has declined. Anthropological research has examined drinking behaviour in many different societies, and shown that disinhibition is by no means a necessary consequence of alcohol consumption despite the well-recognised physiological changes associated with intoxication. Socio-cultural theorists see disinhibition as a product of culture, shaped by an individual's personal concept of drunkenness. This includes his expectation of subsequent behaviour, and is influenced by situational factors such as drinking location, and the attitudes, behaviour and social standing of others present.

As wide-ranging areas of anthropology and sociology have been covered, a highly selective approach is necessary. Research relating specifically to alcohol and aggression has been high-lighted and an attempt made to place it in an appropriate theoretical perspective. Inevitably such approaches have shortcomings. First, it is impossible to adequately describe all the hypotheses referred to in this chapter. Secondly, selection will ignore certain hypotheses of major importance to both criminology and anthropology simply because they have not been examined in relation to alcohol and aggression. Thirdly, an adequate critique of each hypothesis cannot be provided. The more limited aim of this chapter is to provide an overview of areas most relevant to the socio-cultural perspective, and to present an additional approach to the study of alcohol-related aggression for comparison with previous chapters.

Labelling Behaviour As 'Drunken' or 'Aggressive'

Bandura[1] suggested aggression was socially defined on the basis of a variety of factors, many of which reside in the observer and evaluator of the behaviour rather than the performer. Persons of different socio-economic level, sex, ethnic background, educational and occupational status vary in the extent to which they view specific behaviour as drunken or aggressive. Variations in the demographic features of the performer also partly determine whether he receives labels and how he himself perceives them. For example, criminologists have consistently shown that male sex, youth, lower social status, and ethnic minority predispose to arrest and prosecution.[2,3] Stereotypes of drinking behaviour considered socially appropriate are learned by members of society through personal experience and knowledge of cultural norms. Thus, observers may describe an intoxicated individual as having had 'a good drink' when his behaviour is orderly, but 'drunk' when he is disruptive, although the quantity of alcohol consumed may be the same. Similarly, a woman whose bottom is pinched at a drinking party may be unable to persuade observers that she has been the victim of anything other than 'a bit of fun', whereas the same experience in a bus queue might be construed as an assault.

Departures from accepted stereotypes of behaviour or cultural norms may result in an individual being labelled aggressive or disinhibited. However, the mere presence of alcohol can give events a new social meaning. Responses elicited from others, particularly expressions of distress or injury in the recipient, are likely to result in behaviour being labelled aggressive. However, responses can also be redefined in the presence of alcohol. For example, apparent 'over-reaction' by the victim renders the social meaning of the aggressive behaviour as less serious, and the aggressor will be judged less reprehensible. Intentions attributed to the aggressor will further qualify the perceived seriousness, especially if alcohol consumption is thought to reduce the degree to which harm is intended.

Major problems may arise for individuals once they receive the label 'aggressive'. Becker[4] saw society as creating rules whose infraction constituted deviance, with the individual passing through a series of stages until the important point is reached when he is caught and assumes the label or 'master status'. Examples such as 'drunk', 'rapist', 'prostitute' or 'drug-addict' ultimately come to dominate other personal characteristics. Goffman[5] believed that the major problem for the person labelled deviant is to manage such an identity when interacting with others. To cope with the label a process of 'deviance disavowal' is tried — an attempt to sustain oneself as a 'normal' person by verbal justifications and excuses for oneself and one's behaviour involving techniques of 'neutralisation' (see Sykes and Matza[6]). However, some behaviour is particularly hard to justify, and peer group members may view it as so bizarre or despicable they will accept no explanation. The 'deviant' must then either withdraw and accept the label, deny the behaviour, or claim he was virtually powerless to control his behaviour at the time. Alcohol provided an ideal opportunity for the latter strategy in a series of 158 child molesters. McCaghy[7] showed that by claiming intoxication with alcohol these men could substitute a lesser, more acceptable, and temporary deviance for one which was greater and far more challenging to their identity as 'normal' persons. Thus, by emphasising their drinking they could actually admit to deviant behaviour without accepting responsibility for it.

People learn what can be excused in social interactions if they are thought by others to be 'drunk'. Gelles[8] studied married couples between whom there was frequent violence and concluded that men got drunk to have an excuse to beat their wives, rather than becoming violent because they were drunk. This was despite the wives' belief that the drinking constituted the major family problem. In a similar study, Coleman and Strauss[9] demonstrated that as alcohol abuse became extreme, violence actually diminished between spouses, and it occurred as a specific interaction between the spouses rather than towards their children.

Thus, the idea that alcohol releases inhibition by impairing a person's control over his behaviour can become a fundamental part of the social meaning of drinking. Consequently, alcohol-related aggression may be considered less intentional, being the result of pharmacological effects of alcohol rather than reflecting situational factors or personality characteristics of the aggressor. Box[10] points out that 'techniques of neutralisation' can be further reinforced in society by its legal system, giving examples of rapists who received lighter sentences from judges who accepted their excuses of drunkenness. Chapters 5 and 6 have already described how alcohol consumed by rape victims can partly influence the decision-making by criminal justice personnel over whether the offenders are charged and subsequently receive convictions. Furthermore, it may sometimes shift blame for the assault onto the victim herself.

Changes in Social Meaning of Drunkenness Over Time

Levine[11], in an important study of the history of ideas regarding drunkenness in North American society suggested that the social meaning of alcohol as the cause of 'drunken' behaviours such as violence and crime is a relatively recent phenomenon. He believed that many of the ways in which the 'alcohol problem' is currently defined were first articulated only at the beginning of the nineteenth-century. This followed agreement by physicians and laymen associated with the Temperance Movement that alcohol was a dangerous and destructive substance. Earlier contemporary accounts indicated that eighteenth-century American colonials considered alcohol to have primarily good effects, improving health, sociability and making people happy. They did recognise that it could precede or accompany violent or criminal behaviour, but this was exhibited by persons who regularly visited taverns. During the eighteenth-century taverns had become autonomous centres of lower-class social and political life, and their control had moved from the higher social classes who increasingly began to perceive them as potential sources of lower-class disorder. It was not, however, alcohol that was seen as the cause of crime and violence, but the lower-class tavern itself. Religious thinking also had a major influence on contemporary thought, perceiving alcohol as giving access to the devil, and frequent intoxication as evidence of a willingness to do the devil's work. However, settlers did believe that alcohol caused crime and violence among the Indians, and all colonies had laws forbidding the sale of liquor to them. Indians were considered quite different beings from settlers, however; savages were naturally violent in a way that the settlers were not.

By the mid-nineteenth-century a major change in attitude to drinking had gradually taken place. Levine believed this was part of the larger social and economic changes taking place in North American society. Developing capitalism had begun to require greater organisation and discipline from its managers and workers, and produced pressures resulting in a growing preoccupation with maintaining control in both work and family life and facilitating the adoption of abstention. Consumption declined among the higher social classes whereas it increased in the lower stratas of society. The appearance of middle-class 'saloons' enabled men to avoid the stigmatised lower-class taverns, yet get away from their responsibilities and families. Thus, a heavy-drinking, middle-class sub-culture developed, but was stigmatised by respectable members of society. Meanwhile, economic pressures also restricted relaxation time for the working class, and occasions that remained would often involve getting drunk. 'Drinking time' became increasingly associated with the relaxation of controls over behaviour and self-discipline. Thus, in Levine's view, it was likely that a man would have a drink before visiting a prostitute or beating his wife.

Temperance movements of the nineteenth-century developed the most elaborate and convincing image of alcohol as a destructive force and an explanation for social problems such as crime and violence. Wealthy and powerful Americans became increasingly concerned by the effects of liquor on morality, order and worker discipline, and supported the educated and articulate members of the Temperance Movement whom they saw as a countering influence. Overall goals gradually changed from drinking in moderation to total abstention as alcohol was portrayed as the destroyer of self-control, accounting for major social problems, e.g. crime, violence, poverty, business and financial failure. Temperance supporters attempted to demonstrate these propositions with crude statistics showing high percentages of crimes and other social problems after alcohol had been consumed, the implication being that if people did not drink these problems would be eliminated.

Levine's analysis is of major importance to the socio-cultural perspective because it implies that the social meaning of drinking behaviour can undergo major change with time. Furthermore, changes for the worse are clearly to be anticipated from specific social groups, such as Indians and the lower social classes, over whom control must by necessity be re-established. The study also indicates that these changes in ideas were linked to the need for change in social behaviour following industrial development. Parallels can be drawn with the introduction of licensing hours in Britain during the 1914-18 war, when workers' drinking was considered to have impaired their industrial output essential for the war effort.

Mass Media Influences

Winick[12] highlights the importance of the mass media as an influence on cultural beliefs in Western society, claiming that in the USA the average adult spends more time in contact with various forms of media than he does in working or sleeping. However, it is unclear from his survey whether the wide range of drinking stereotypes portrayed in literature, newspapers, popular music, films and on television are actually shaping current ideas and introducing new influences, or whether the media reflects those already present in society. One important observation is an apparent increase in sheer numbers of alcohol-related events portrayed, shown most strikingly in studies of prime time television where 80 per cent of programmes involve some reference to alcoholic beverage, with an average of two acts of alcohol-use an hour. Drinking behaviour is most frequently portrayed as a way to relax, cope with a problem, or be sophisticated. Alcohol-related disinhibition is by no means typical. Stereotypes of alcohol and violence range from saloon brawls in westerns to secret agents who always remain cool and in control, dispatching villains with a revolver in one hand and a glass in the other. Winick did observe a repetitive stereotype in television 'soap operas' where characters suffering personal disappointments or failure respond with a bout of heavy drinking and disinhibited behaviour subsequently regretted. Overall, however, the US media does not routinely convey the message that alcohol leads to disinhibited behaviour, according to Winick's review. Media influences appear more involved in 'normalising' drinking behaviour in society (with implications for consumption level rather than disinhibition), portraying it as a regular and expected part of social interaction. Advertising techniques reinforce this by ignoring drinking problems and associating drink with wealth, prestige and success, social approval, relaxation and leisure, exotic locations, individualistic behaviour, and sex.

Distortion of public attitudes by unbalanced presentation of news events has been an area of major interest to criminologists. The ability of the media to create a phenomenon of violence by the process of 'Deviance Amplification' has been described in a study of community reaction to the 'mods and rockers' in Britain in the 1960s.[13] Minor incidents had attracted considerable media attention, and violence and damage were greatly exaggerated. Youngsters were simplistically grouped into 'mods' or 'rockers' according to their style of dress, with a subsequent self-fulfilling identification of young people in stereotyped rival groups. Over subsequent weekends, increasing numbers of young people travelled to seaside towns seeking excitement in belonging to these youth movements, having been provided with stereotypes of appropriate behaviour and dress by the media. Local communities sensitised to expect trouble reacted in a hostile manner, and local magistrates and police reacted punitively. Hostility was reciprocated by hooligans who revelled in increasing media attention and dramatisation of their behaviour.

Further studies of media coverage of violence show that what constitutes the 'news' for any one day is highly selected from a large number of potential items and presented in a specific way. For example, Winick was struck by an apparent lack of alcohol involvement in violent crimes reported in US newspapers, in marked contrast to police impressions. Thus, 'news' is an entity created by editors and journalists. Chibnall[14] studied crime reporting in the British press and noted the small number of journalists actually involved in creating news stories across the country, observing certain patterns which underlie their method of story construction. Descriptions always tended to report immediate happenings rather than processes unfolding more slowly. Only sufficient background material to make events intelligible at a mundane level. Dramatisation was achieved by stressing stories with impact, and the individuals involved were given simplistic 'characters'. Novelty was essential, with attempts to gain new angles often leading to speculation based on the slenderest of evidence. Vicarious titillations and gossip were provided whilst the newspaper studiously distanced itself from the activities portrayed. Meanwhile, journalists took the stance that they were professionals and merely reporting the facts, their articles frequently imbued with the pronouncement of 'experts'. For example, an article entitled 'How Drinkers Turn to Rape and Murder' in a major British newspaper in 1980 clearly illustrates several of the features observed by Chibnall. The dramatic headline suggests that drinkers risk becoming rapists and murderers and that an epidemic of such behaviour could be underway. The journalist claimed to be uncertain how this process took place, and the article gradually merged into a somewhat irrelevant report of prisoners paroled — Lord Harris and the Parole Board were introduced as the necessary 'experts' to lend authority to the piece. The journalist expressed bewilderment that Britian was 'only eighth' in the beer-drinking league, behind New Zealand and Denmark, countries not noted for their high rates of murder and rape.

Clearly, the media can portray alcohol-related behaviours as of greater or lesser seriousness, sometimes engendering anxiety in the public. Articles such as that cited above are unlikely to influence many in this way, but do illustrate the media's potential to create a generalised set of beliefs 'explaining' complex behaviours such as murder and rape. Blame can be spuriously attributed to alcohol where there is little evidence of a direct association, and the public can be sensitised to anticipate deviant behaviour in certain drinking locations. Images are created by headlines such as 'drunken animals' to describe football hooligans suggest their is no human rationale behind their action.[15] Simplistic explanations such as irrational collective spasms or temporary alcohol-induced insanity ignore the other social conflicts and antagonisms such as poverty, unemployment and racism that may be of greater importance. Confirmation of these stereotypes by the media leads to a greater emphasis on the need for social control of drinking, and the application of severe penalties to individuals who behave aggressively when drinking, rather than examining the social problems contributing to this behaviour.

Learning Drinking and Aggressive Behaviour

Haralambos[16] describes culture as both learned and shared, and such an integral part of society that its members are often unaware of it. The process of learning culture takes place from childhood through socialisation within the family, peer group, educational system, occupational group, and will be influenced by external agencies such as advertising and the media. Human aggression includes patterns of behaviour that are acquired through direct experience or the observation of others, and is learnt through differential reinforcement. However, certain anthropologists[17] have indicated that not all societies are aggressive. Indeed, within some apparently aggressive non-literate societies the behaviour between members is mainly non-aggressive. Among these people the child-rearing practices are characterised by the reward of co-operative behaviour and discouragement of aggression, with adults setting models for children to imitate. The high level of child care results in their learning to accept limitations on their behaviour as they grow older, aided by adults other than their parents in taking responsibility for unacceptable behaviour. Cultural beliefs frequently define hostile feelings as unwanted and unhealthy, and violence between members is seen as due to lack of control and a matter for shame. Societies that foster the opposite values and norms of behaviour, and employ contrasting methods of child-rearing, are characterised by high levels of intra-group violence. Chapter 6 has already outlined evidence suggesting that these societies are characterised by higher levels of intra- and inter-group violence towards women. Unfortunately, there is a dearth of studies that have specifically examined drinking behaviour according to childhood socialisation patterns, necessitating looking at the development of aggressive and drinking behaviours separately.

Plant[18] describes the process of learning to drink and associated behaviour as developing through socialisation. Young children in Glasgow were able to recognise drunken behaviour in a film, and by the age of 8 years had mastered the concept of alcohol and associated it with undesirable behaviour, often witnessed in their own homes or neighbourhoods.[19] Children of the same age showed a critical understanding of aggressive behaviour, the situations in which it is most likely to occur, and the appraisals and emotions concomitant with it.[20] Sex stereotyping was seen for both drinking and aggressive behaviour, with Glaswegian boys being given more encouragement to sample beer by their parents than were girls. Furthermore, by the age of 6 years both boys and girls believed that boys were more likely to see situations as provocative, get angry, be unable to restrain anger once aroused, and also express anger as aggression. This consensus was even stronger among older children. Thus, although the exact nature of the early social experience necessary for a concept of drink-related aggression remains unclear, it is likely to involve drunken assaults between parents or older siblings, or be witnessed by the children within their neighbourhood or on TV. In all cases, males were generally aggressors.

By their teens, children are no longer influenced to the same degree by their families. In a second Glaswegian study the earlier negative attributes for drinking were observed to change to new stereotypes of drinkers as sociable and tough, and abstainers as weak and unsociable.[21] By 17 years, the peer group is firmly established as the main influence, leading to increasing drinking. Young people observe their friends drinking, a behaviour now considered socially desirable, prestigious and an indication of maturity. Plant observed that by the time adulthood was reached, the individual would drink according to social circumstances and would pass through fairly clear-cut 'drinking careers'. The majority of young persons becoming heavily involved are young males from socially deprived backgrounds having a multiplicity of social and psychological problems. In contrast, women and middle-class persons drink less and have fewer alcohol-related problems. Most young alcohol abusers decrease their consumption as they find jobs or develop other interests, and particularly when they marry. Plant believed these influences steer them away from the heavy-drinking peer group. Continuing heavy drinkers are likely to be part of a social group where these patterns of consumption are the norm, or else in a higher-risk occupation with ready availability of liquor and encouragement to consume it.

Similarities are apparent in follow-up studies of delinquent behaviour.[22 to 25] In the early and middle 20s there is a decline in antisocial behaviour; many juvenile offenders cease to be delinquent. Again, factors such as taking a job, stable marriage to non-delinquent partners, and moving to a new neighbourhood away from the delinquent peer group, correlate with these changes. In West's[26] study of teenage youths in a working-class area of London, aggression was frequent, with a majority of the boys having regular fights and many carrying weapons. However, in terms of convictions, the most aggressive individuals came from large, poor families with criminal members. In addition, they had shown persisting traits of aggressiveness from an early age, with higher levels of disruptive behaviour both at school and at home. The more factors that accumulated of both individual traits and disadvantageous environmental influence, the more persistent their criminal (including violent) behaviour in adulthood. Thus, the general notion that mixing with others who drink heavily, behave aggressively, and commit delinquent acts leading to similar behaviour, receives some support from empirical research.

Anthropological Studies of Drunken Comportment

In 1969, Craig MacAndrew and Robert B. Edgerton published an anthropological study of drunken behaviour in different societies.[27] Their work was seminal, focusing attention away from alcohol's 'internal' (mediated through biochemical and physiological mechanisms) effects and onto the external influences of the society of which the individual is a member. By surveying the previous research in a wide range of pre-industrial and tribal societies, they demonstrated a wide repertoire of drinking behaviour in different locations and the same locations over time. The main finding was that violence and promiscuity were by no means inevitable consequences of drinking. Six major phenomena demonstrating how socio-cultural influences largely determine behaviour when a person is intoxicated may be summarised from their work.

(1) *Certain Societies Fail to Exhibit Disinhibition*

In a wide range of Indian tribes in North and South America, some were found to exhibit 'changes for the worse' after drinking whereas others did not. In Britain a simple contrast might be drawn between drinking behaviours of different social classes stereotyped in the comportment observed in Glaswegian public houses compared with the Pall Mall gentlemen's club.

(2) *Time and Circumstances of Drinking Affect Behaviour*

There are societies whose members' drunken behaviour is radically different from one set of socially ordered situations to another. For example, the Maori were described as having different drinking situations termed 'parties' or 'sessions' when young persons of different sexes would meet. At parties there would be fighting and promiscuity, whereas at 'sessions' the participants would talk and fall asleep. Similarly, the Papago tribe considered the use of their words for 'drunkenness' and 'dizzy' after drinking to be sacred and poetic, although this did not always apply to their drinking behaviour, as one particular tribe's drinking ceremonies eventually gave way with time to brawling and violence. The presence of key persons appears important in determining behaviour in different situations. For example, the Taira of Japan never exhibited aggression when men and women drank together, but fights would break out when the men drank by themselves.

(3) *Drunken Comportment is Limited by Social Controls*

Drunkenness is not a state where all sense of right and wrong is lost, and when detrimental changes do occur they are usually within the limits expected by society. Thus, with rare exceptions, there are limits beyond which even the most seemingly disinhibited drunkard will not go, implying that a considerable degree of social control continues to be exerted. These rare exceptions are often labelled as 'sick', and can attract psychiatric diagnoses to explain the behaviour.[28]

(4) *Specificity of Target for Drunken Aggression*

Early reports by missionaries (and recent descriptions by anthropologists living with frequently drunk and violent Indians) have noted that they were virtually never assaulted themselves. In addition, some tribes would fight among themselves during drinking bouts, but the men would never assault their wives who waited on them (the opposite has also been observed). MacAndrew and Edgerton[27] concluded that when drunkenness is accompanied by the relaxation of normally operating rules for behaviour, 'selectivity' of object is usually observed for both sexual and aggressive behaviour. In most cases the object for assault is an equal in status or a perceived inferior, although the Abipone, for example, would sometimes take the opportunity of drinking bouts to settle scores with their chiefs.

(5) *Time Out*

In some cultures drunkenness is a state which is socially sanctioned as free from the constraints of the law. In others, specific times such as religious ceremonies and fiestas are set aside when drunken behaviour is tolerated. Here drunkenness is 'time out' from the otherwise imperative demands on an individual's everyday behaviour by society. Of course, the true contribution of the drinking varies widely when examined more closely. Drunkenness will be quite incidental to certain special occasions when 'time out' behaviour occurs — sometimes in the total absence of alcohol.

(6) *Drunken Behaviour Changes Over Time*

In certain societies drunken behaviour undergoes major changes over time. The Tahitians were recorded to express distaste for alcohol when first exposed to it, but showed widespread drunkenness when they finally accepted it and then more amiable drinking patterns and sociable behaviour over time. Similarly, Marshall[29] believed that drunken brawling became a substitute to maintain the 'machismo' ethic for Micronesian males after warfare had been prohibited. Studies of North American Indians have also detailed changes in drunken behaviour with time. Laws forbidding sale of liquor to Indians existed for many years, but MacAndrew and Edgerton[27] believed their first encounters with alcohol were not affected by expectations of subsequent behaviour. In addition, the all-consuming craving, drunken mayhem and debauchery later considered typical of drunken Indians was not initially observed.

These authors hypothesised that white men provided a model for drunken behaviour, and by observation Indians also learnt that drink would excuse behaviour, citing examples of Indians who feigned drunkenness before committing murder.

Coping with the Introduction of Alcohol into Society

Feest[30] believes that positive integration of alcohol and culture is more likely when consumers and producers are the same. Many of the extreme problems encountered by North American Indians were thought to stem from their not producing their own liquor, but depending on importation from an alien culture. Problems were further exacerbated by the pressure to consume exerted by profit-motivated white traders. Introduction of alcohol *de novo* provides an important opportunity to examine how less advanced societies attempt to cope with the potentially disastrous effects on their members' behaviour. Feest has observed two major processes that temporarily controlled the adverse effects of drinking in Indian societies.

(a) *Active Integration.* Customs emerged in certain tribes which specified the purpose, frequency, and consequences of drinking, containing individual's drinking behaviour according to the norms of society. Alcohol, in these cases, actually strengthened social bonds, reduced tensions, and provided socially redeeming purposes. These societies tolerated alcohol intoxication by channelling it and integrating it. However, any deviation from culturally defined and socially approved patterns of alcohol-use had to be stigmatised. For example, the Creeks and Seminoles showed severe societal disruption in the initial stages of encountering alcohol. Later, they not only came to accept alcohol, but stressed the positive aspects of communal drinking. Concomitantly, provisions were made to safeguard against further disintegrative tendencies from the unrestricted drinking of tribal members. It was these *informal* methods of social control which ultimately proved more effective than unenforceable laws. Legal sanctions applied by the white man had little effect on Indian drinking patterns, and the more coercive effects of informal sanctions are reflected in the law's failure to regulate drunken behaviour in Western society.

(b) *Ideological Rejection.* Certain tribes to varying degrees and for varying lengths of time rejected alcohol for what were ideological reasons. Revitalisation movements such as the 'Dream Dance' and natavistic movements such as the Peyote religion successfully controlled drinking problems for some tribes, as the doctrines of these new religions and movements contained the rejection of alcohol consumption. For example, the Comanche consisted of loosely integrated bands of hunters whom one might have expected to have a predisposition heavy drinking, possibly involving problem behaviour. Historical descriptions show that initial offers of alcohol by white men were rejected for reasons which remain unclear to anthropologists. Later, these barriers were eroded, and alcohol accepted with 'typical' drunken Indian behaviour of violence, mayhem, and social disintegration, exacerbated by wholesale exploitation by white traders. The subsequent development of the Peyote cult represented a new ideology against drinking, and (while it lasted) alcohol was again rejected by the Comanches. Parallels can be drawn with religious movements and organisations in Western society, such as Alcoholics Anonymous. There are, however, a wide range of organisations, and adherence to their principles is not as uniform as is possible in a tribal society.

Purpose and Ritualisation in Drunken Aggression

Theories of social deviations serving an important function for society have a long history. Durkheim[31] maintained they serve to define and reinforce moral boundaries of acceptable and non-acceptable behaviour by social sanction and criminalisation. Violations of certain norms result in harsh reactions, whilst other transgressions produce little or no reaction. Individuals sufficiently integrated into group and community life are socialised to accept its traditional or dominant values and become norm-abiding members. Deviants are assumed to be inadequately socialised. Merton[32] distinguished between 'manifest' and 'latent' functions in society. Manifest functions are objective consequences contributing to the adaptation of the system which are both intended and recognised: latent functions are neither intended or recognised. Thus, what may at first appear dysfunctional may be otherwise, and vice versa.

Horton[33] proposed that alcohol's primary *function* in society was to reduce anxiety. The larger the consumption, the more completely anxiety would be reduced. The greater the anxiety, the more alcohol is required to reduce it. To Horton, drinking behaviour is a state of dynamic equilibrium with anxiety-reduction providing the chief motivation, and anticipation of punishments for unacceptable behaviour being the chief counteracting factor. Field[34] re-examined Horton's theory and confirmed that primitive hunting and gathering societies tended to have more drunkenness than agricultural economies. He suggested, however, that this was not due to higher levels of anxiety, but to the social organisation within these societies.

More recent commentaries on cultural patterns of alcohol-related aggression also emphasise functional aspects of drinking but admit that social organisation acts simultaneously. Levinson[35] summarised function in two ways: (i) 'Drive Discharge' — the concept that all individuals and social groups have a certain level of innate aggression that must be periodically discharged; and (ii) 'Cultural Defence Mechanisms' — the concept that drunken aggression reduces anxiety, tension and insecurity. He saw the association between drinking patterns and alcohol-related problems as depending largely on the extent to which alcohol use is integrated into the sub-cultural system. Social structure and social control were seen as essential prerequisites. More highly structured societies emphasised authority and respect in their interpersonal relationships, with consequent controlled drinking behaviour.

Marshall's[29] study of drinking on the Micronesian island of Truk also conforms to the Functionalist approach. He warned against assumptions that drunken, rowdy and disruptive behaviour necessarily implied a severe breakdown in society's functioning. Apparently deviant behaviour (to the outsider) may be a normal and culturally sanctioned pattern for coping with stress and the tensions of life. Within specific cultural, legal and ideological conditions, drunkenness and brawling may be no more deviant than total sobriety, pent-up aggression, and compulsive work habits as modes of adapting to cultural change. On Truk, getting drunk appeared an affirmation of cultural continuity rather than disintegration. Virtually all men aged 18-35 years engaged in weekly drinking bouts accompanied by frequent outbursts of violence, usually directed at youths from other villages. In Truk society it was considered deviant not to get drunk, as young men were expected to behave aggressively, prove their manliness, take risks, and engage in amorous pursuits. Marshall believed that drunkenness was their means of venting pent-up aggression, often related to feelings of powerlessness concerning other aspects of their island life. Drunken brawling appeared to have become the means of expressing these feelings when warfare was prohibited.

An important question remains concerning the extent to which drunken behaviour is truly socially controlled. Marshall's work suggests a degree of 'rule-following' behaviour on Truk, where young men were required to behave in different ways on different occasions, particularly with respect to their elders. To some extent, their drunken behaviour could be considered 'ritualised', with unwritten rules governing the permitted degree of aggression, to whom they could direct the behaviour, and where and when they could be aggressive. Marsh[36] and Marsh, Rosser and Harre[37] believe that societies create and maintain social controls on the extent and nature of violence, developing rituals that contain it and allow safe expression. Studying soccer violence in Britain, they saw hooligans as expressing a need to identify with a highly distinctive group. Fighting at football matches appeared to Marsh to be within defined limits of social conventions and constraints amongst the fans. Displays of hostility, conventions of challenge and counter-challenge were much more apparent than actual violence — an observation which applies to warfare in small, non-literate societies.[17] Unfortunately, there is little information on alcohol's influence on soccer hooliganism despite official policies to ban its sale at football grounds. Further research may examine whether drinking patterns amongst supporters before a match are part of their ritualisation of violence, such as giving 'dutch courage', or reaffirming group cohesion by drinking together. In contrast, alcohol might also loosen the constraints on 'rule-following' behaviour in some individuals, sometimes to the extent of inflicting particularly severe injuries on their rivals.

Theories of Alcohol-related Violence in Western Urban Settings

Increasing development and industrialisation have left few tribal societies in isolation, and increasingly presents them with the problems of Western society. Anthropologists have therefore increasingly turned to studies of more complex societies.[38] With the routine collection of statistics it has become possible to compare rates of social problems, including crimes of violence and alcohol-related morbidity and mortality, according to residential area. Methodological problems arise through variations in definition of measured problems and the many deficiencies of official statistics.[39] Furthermore, the geographical patterns found are merely the spatial outcome of a complex of social processes which require further explanation. However, epidemiological studies of urban environments do provide a useful reference point from which to formulate some of the major socio-cultural theories relating to alcohol and aggressive behaviour.

A considerable literature links urbanisation and the growth of cities with increasing rates of crime.[40] Criminologists have taken particular interest in urban environments since the 1920s, when sociologists under the direction of Robert Park developed a major research project in Chicago. Urban growth appeared to occur through zones which developed in concentric rings from the centre outwards. Growth was not a random process, but orderly and predictable, being influenced by successive waves of immigrants to the city. Five typical zones were recognised as Chicago developed around the central business district, which was surrounded by the second zone in 'transition', characterised by encroachment of industry and older deteriorating housing — the area where immigrants first lived before progressing to outer zones with increasing economic success. The three outer zones housed first the stable working class, the middle classes, and most peripherally the outer ring of wealthy suburbs and dormitory areas. An ecological theory of crime was developed linking deviant behaviour to particular conditions in the zone in transition. It must be emphasised that this positivistic theory ignored 'white-collar' crime, but official statistics showed that the transition zone had the highest rates of especially violent crime, with a progressive fall moving to the outer zone. It also housed the highest proportion of mentally ill, alcoholics, overcrowded and low-income families, and had the poorest educational, recreational and policing provisions. No matter which ethnic group moved in, levels of deviance remained high, leading researchers to conclude that factors relating to the natural areas themselves rather than the populations in them led to the deviance. Further research showed a high mobility within the transitional zone, resulting in particularly unstable social relationships between residents, characterised by impersonalism, distrust, suspicion, and lack of social support.

The classic 'concentric ring' model is less appropriate to most British cities, where the local authority housing estate is considered by criminologists[41] to be the most appropriate phenomenon in the ecological tradition. Local authorities may contribute to this phenomenon by allocating the worst accommodation to coloured immigrants[42] and 'problem families'[43] creating so-called 'dump' estates.[44] Murray and Boal[45] reviewed British studies of violent crime according to residential area, confirming the association with high levels of other social problems. Violence was more likely within or in the locality of the offender's home. When, however, attacks on strangers were specifically examined they tended to relate to the geographical location of public houses. In their review, the authors outlined eight different sociological phenomena potentially explaining intraurban variations in violence. This framework is not restricted by narrowly concentrating on an environmental approach to the exclusion of others, and is a useful reference point from which to examine alcohol-related violence in the urban setting. The phenomena were as follows.

(a) *Differential Opportunity.* Certain types of microenvironment have higher rates of violence because they present more opportunities for disputes to arise. Intraurban variations in violence are consequently due to the distribution of such locations. Lambert[46] examined a sector of Birmingham, and McClintock, Avison, Savill and Worthington[47] a sector of London, using police sub-divisions as the area unit. They found that incidents of violence were relatively rare events, most cases arising from domestic disputes or arguments in the street or public house associated with alcohol. Lambert's study specifically showed that the occurrence of violent incidents arising from street disturbances is closely related to the distributions of public houses. It is surprising that these findings have not provided the focus for more studies in Britain, particularly as certain drinking locations can become notorious both to local people and the police. Fortunately, there is a small amount of North American data on bars that are characterised by deviant behaviour. Graham, LaRocque, Yetmann, Ross and Guistra[48] studied 185 drinking establishments in Vancouver, and showed that aggression was highly predictable on the basis of situational variables. The most violence-prone bars were in skid-row districts, had permissive decorum expectations, and unpleasant, unsanitary and inexpensive physical surroundings. There was a higher incidence of American Indians and unkempt patrons, and the atmosphere tended to be tense, with patrons drinking rapidly, becoming highly intoxicated, and with people talking loudly to themselves.

(b) *Differential Drift.* This assumes there are people who already have violence-prone lifestyles or personalities. Rejected or unable to live in most other areas, they tend to drift to the inner city. As has already been described, housing allocation policies can contribute to such individuals being grouped together in certain geographical locations. Graham's Vancouver study did not examine this factor in great detail, but her findings are broadly consistent with the notion that socially deprived, disorganised and difficult individuals who had in various ways been excluded from others, had found bars with permissive expectations of appearance and behaviour. Burns[49] demonstrated that certain individuals will temporarily visit certain drinking locations to behave in a disinhibited fashion — a process which is not quite the same as 'differential drift'. Describing a night out with a group of young men in Charlestown, Boston, he observed that aggressive behaviour whilst drinking depended on location. Polite and deferential behaviour was shown to older, more stable members of their own local community in a neighbourhood 'family' bar where they started drinking at the beginning of their night out. Once outside, however, and on the way to more exciting locations, the young men began to exhibit mildly aggressive behaviour directed at each other, jostling in an increasingly rowdy manner. Later that evening they exhibited their most aggressive behaviour towards strangers and prostitutes drinking in a bar in Boston's downtown 'Combat Zone'. One became involved in an argument with a stranger, another was involved in breaking a window, and the third (and rowdiest) was threatened with a gun. On the way home, they narrowly escaped arrest. Within their home neighbourhood such behaviour would not be tolerated, and it was the excitement of a permissive environment where prostitutes, drug-use, heavy drinking, and alcohol-related violence could be found that attracted them to the final location.

(c) *Violent Sub-culture.* In certain geographical areas, or within certain groups living within these areas, a sub-culture may develop which rejects the majority culture and its values. Instead, it encourages, or at least condones, the use of violence as a legitimate form of behaviour. Thus, members who engage in violence may simply be acting in a normal fashion. Studies of sub-culture and alcohol-related violence have concentrated mainly on the 'sub-culture of violence' theory.[50] This section will restrict itself to this narrow facet of the otherwise complex and wide-ranging sub-cultural perspective of deviant behaviour.

Wolfgang and Ferracuti[50] believed that certain populations have different attitudes towards the use of violence reflected in their criminal statistics. They provided anthropological evidence that cultures with the highest rates of homicide have particularly accepting attitudes to sudden, violent death within sub-sections of their communities. In his earlier study of criminal homicide in Philadelphia, Wolfgang[51] found that 60 per cent of offenders had been drinking before the crime. Alcohol-related homicide was more frequent at weekends, holidays, pay-days, and between the hours of 8 p.m. and 2 a.m. Both participants were likely to be males who had been drinking together, although alcohol was frequently associated with domestic altercations in which a female sexual partner was killed. Thus, drinking tended to occur in close interpersonal interactions, particularly in social, emotional, and/or competitive situations. A larger proportion of offenders were black, there was a strong statistical association with the lowest social class, and weapons were often used that were regularly carried by these men. Alcohol was associated with an extreme degree of violence inflicted upon the victim in terms of the number of blows, shots or stabs received. The victims themselves had usually been drinking, often more than the offender when two males were involved — a factor Wolfgang believed may have determined the participant who was finally killed. Not surprisingly 'victim-precipitation' (where the victim has provoked his own death) was a frequent finding. However, rather than attributing these results to pharmacological effects, Wolfgang stressed the drinking situation and the lifestyles of his intoxicated subjects. Heavy drinking and the acceptance of violence as legitimate means of settling differences in the poorest parts of Philadelphia, particularly the Ghetto, were considered major explanations for his findings.

Roizen[52] has reviewed the literature on crime and drinking by blacks, and rejected the idea that negroes are more likely to be involved in alcohol-related crimes if social class is controlled for. However, certain black drinking contexts such as ghetto taverns are important locations for planning and carrying out criminal activities. These taverns are also social centres for lower-class blacks where drinking serves utilitarian and escape functions. Clientele sometimes include a particularly deviant sub-group, many of whom have drunk heavily from an early age and who have long criminal histories. In certain taverns the setting is legitimate for personal confrontations and violence, with a general freedom from the behavioural norms of everyday life. Some patrons have a propensity for violence, and in many cases have little to lose from its occurrence. Roizen insists that frequenters of ghetto taverns should not be considered representative of blacks in general, and that drinking patterns, subsequent aggressive behaviour, and other drinking problems do not show major differences when social class is controlled for.

(d) *Social Alienation.* The residents of certain areas, particularly if they belong to a minority ethnic group or some underclass, are alienated from society, leading to feelings of powerlessness and hostility increasing the likelihood of violence. This important theory has not been examined specifically in relation to alcohol and aggression.

(e) *Stress.* When demands made on an individual or group exceed their resources, either due to inadequacies in their resources or excessive demands, persons under these stresses are more likely to resort to violence. Such stresses are particularly marked in deprived urban areas. Lewis[53] recorded a tendency to 'live for the moment' and not to plan for the future among the poor in cities such as New York, Lima and Mexico City. This seems a rational response to conditions of powerlessness and poverty, which once in existence tend to be perpetuated. Harrison[44] observed similar processes in Hackney, London, and believed that perpetuation of social problems over time was not merely because the people living there were less efficient at managing their incomes or inherently prone to solving problems in limited ways. Rather, the stresses of being poor and the consequent lack of alternative strategies appeared of greater importance in maintaining patterns of behaviour. This view did not examine in detail the relation between alcohol and violent behaviour, but appears an important area with scope for future research. It might be argued that drinking patterns and problems in situations of deprivation facilitate inappropriate strategies aimed at coping, but which further increase stress suffered by these individuals and their families.

(f) *Frustration/Relative Deprivation.* Frustration occurs when individuals or groups are prevented from satisfying some need they expect to gratify. This hypothesis is largely derived from Merton's[32] postulate of a state of conflict of norms regarding goals for individuals in society, and the means of achieving them when the accepted methods are largely blocked. Deviant behaviour was seen as a response to blocked access to the accepted goals of society. Citing the USA, Merton saw money, material possessions, status and power emphasised as the goals, but without provision of the means for everyone to achieve them.

Robbins[54] examined drinking patterns of Naspaki men in Canada, interpreting their behaviour as enabling them to maintain and protect their individual social identities. Two types of drinker were described according to subsequent behaviour, which Robbins attributed to differences in their access to status-conferring goods. 'Friendly drunks' were men who earned good wages as iron miners, and where the drinking behaviour maintained and reinforced their high social status. Aggressive drinkers were assertive, boastful, got into fights and were unable to hold jobs as miners. Robbins saw their drinking as an attempt to maintain an old identity threatened by new economic processes. Lurie[55] and others have, however, rejected the idea that heavy drinking by Indians is due to their blocked access to the goals of white society.

(g) *Disorganisation.* One view of aggressive behaviour is that it is due to the fragmentation of the usual bonds between people that society depends on for its persistence and stability. These processes and their disorganisation by alcohol and disinhibited problem behaviour have already been described in some detail.

(h) *Differential Policing/Labelling.* Levels of violence in different residential areas are based on official statistics. These reflect the reputations of certain areas and the individuals living there. Consequently, they are often subjected to more intense police scrutiny. Interactions between groups with very different perceptions, especially youths from inner-city areas and the police, are likely to result in violent incidents.[56] Differential treatment of blacks and whites could partly account for different rates of alcohol-related criminal convictions in these populations, and certain drinking locations could at times be singled out for close police observation. Specific research designed to test these hypotheses in relation to alcohol and violence is presently lacking.

Limitations of the Socio-cultural Perspective

Professionals dealing directly with aggressive drunks and their victims may find it difficult to accept that such disinhibited behaviour follows 'rules', fulfils an important function for society, or is in some way a product of labelling. Indeed, it must be asked whether socio-cultural theories sometimes minimise the damage and distress caused by problem behaviour after drinking by rationalising and searching for meaning. Berkowitz[57] points out that theories of rule-following aggression tend to ignore the distinction between instrumental and hostile (or angry) aggression. These components are not easily separated, in particular incidents which generally involve a combination of expressive, hostile and instrumental features. Although some incidents appear to partially follow rules (particularly group assaults), the individual participants frequently experience high levels of internal excitation, and later report not being in control or failing to think of the consequences. Indeed, the expression of anger and relief of intense emotion may sometimes involve injury to the victim, and these aspects of violent assault may be exacerbated by alcohol.

Room[58] has claimed that modern ethnography has systematically underestimated a wide range of alcohol-related problems. He noted that studies published before 1930 were more likely to report extreme insobriety and regular drunken brawling. Impressions from research can be distorted through methodological artifacts, such as paradigms which under- or over-estimate individual factors, and the interpretation of data where these measurements are 'played up', 'played down', or just ignored. Room believed that all three interpretational errors have occurred in anthropological research, but that 'deflation' of alcohol-related problems has been more apparent in recent years in contrast with pre-1930 findings. Several factors were thought to account for this. Room perceived a strong Functionalist influence in recent literature which tends to ignore drinking at the individual level, focusing instead on stabilising, pattern-maintaining processes in the social life of communities studied. Implicit in this image of society is the assumption that drinking patterns created within, according to customary patterns, are 'good', whereas drinking behaviour derived from external influences is 'bad', as it disrupts social organisation. Room believed these assumptions result in an over-emphasis of gains rather than losses from drinking. In addition, the pleasures of drinking are more easily observed in anthropological studies of everyday life, rather than in the alcohol-related morbidity and mortality which are the focus of the epidemiologist. English-speaking and North American researchers have dominated the alcohol ethnography literature over the last 50 years and Room believes these workers reacted to the perceived narrow-mindedness and moralism of the later Temperance movements, and have been committed to an alternative middle-class ideal of 'moderate drinking'. However, he feels that in the new generation of alcohol ethnographers (often working within their own societies) problem amplification may become more common.

Psychological research into alcohol-related disinhibition is increasingly aligned with socio-cultural theory. Reviews of experimental findings suggest that aggressive, sexual and social disinhibition are primarily a product of *expectancy* that alcohol has been consumed regardless of actual content, with the assumption that expectancy is the direct result of cultural influence.[59,60] Few would argue that culture and circumstances largely determine the interpretation of subjective feelings of intoxication and the way they are acted on by the majority of individual drinkers. However, biological and pharmacological effects still cannot be entirely dismissed. In his review of experimental psychological literature, Lang[59] concedes that very high doses, or alcohol interacting with particular physiological predisposition such as brain abnormality, could precipitate disinhibited behaviour in certain individuals. Furthermore, most psychological research has been on 'normal' populations, usually college students, and seldom with the higher quantities of alcohol that are consumed by those who have committed serious crimes of violence when intoxicated. Psychological research has not extensively examined the pharmacological effects of alcohol on cognition and emotion in relation to the highly complex social interactions terminating in aggression. These alternative psychological processes may be quite independent of both expectancy and cultural influence. Lessons can be drawn from delinquency research where individual trait and environmental theories are no longer in opposition.[2]

Conclusion

From a narrowly defined socio-cultural viewpoint, aggressive behaviour is not an inevitable consquence of drinking, which when it does occur, is precipitated by external circumstances. At the individual level such behaviour is determined largely by attitudes towards and expectations of subsequent behaviour, and therefore conforms to cultural norms of drinking behaviour. Children in most societies learn what to expect from drinking at an early age, and observe that the mere presence of alcohol can lend a new social meaning to aggressive interactions in certain situations, providing an excuse for behaviour that would otherwise not be tolerated. Aggressive behaviour is also learnt during socialisation and profoundly influenced by child-rearing patterns (see Bandura[1], Montagu[17], Feldman[61] for more detailed analysis than provided above). Alcohol-related aggression thus tends to occur in a society, or sub-group within a larger society, that tolerates it and/or encourages it. Violent behaviour (both drunken and sober) is most likely to be exhibited by young males of the lowest social class with a previous history of difficult behaviour, often coming from ethnic and under-privileged minorities. Incidents recorded as alcohol-related violence occur most frequently in run-down bars in deprived inner-city areas that house persons with the highest rates of social problems. Non alcohol-related violence and criminal behaviour are also more frequent in these areas, and several socio-cultural theoretical explanations have been presented to account for these findings.

However, certain drinking locations tolerate a particularly disorganised, inadequate, and/or criminal sub-group of persons whose lifestyles frequently involve various forms of deviant behaviour, including violence.[62] Among these individuals are persons who do not conform to prevailing norms of drinking behaviour and who do not in any way 'belong' to a deviant sub-culture. Socio-cultural theory cannot explain all forms of deviant behaviour, and factors such as individual personality traits, varying physiological response to alcohol, and psychiatric abnormality, will also be necessary to explain certain alcohol-related disinhibition. Furthermore, even apparently normal individuals occasionally exhibit violent behaviour over which they have little control, and which cannot be satisfactorily explained by situational context or cultural norms and expectations. Clearly, problems will arise when attempting to build up a comprehensive picture of the association between alcohol and aggression if socio-cultural and psychological perspectives are over-stated and emphasised to the exclusion of pharmacological and physiological components.

Acknowledgement

I would like to thank Pat Carlen and Angela Burr for their advice on the manuscript.

References

1. Bandura, A. *Aggression: A Social Learning Analysis*, Englewood Cliffs, New Jersey: Prentice-Hall Inc., 1973.
2. Rutter, M. and Giller, H. *Juvenile Delinquency: Trends and Perspectives*, Harmondsworth, Middlesex: Penguin Books, 1983.
3. Smith, D.A., Visher, C.A. and Davidson, L.A. 'Equity and discretionary justice: the influence of race on police arrest decisions', *Journal of Criminal Law and Criminology*, 1984, *75*, 234-49.
4. Becker, H. *Outsiders*, New York: Free Press, 1971.
5. Goffman, E. *Stigma: Notes on the Management of Spoiled Identity*, Englewood Cliffs, New Jersey: Prentice-Hall Inc., 1963.
6. Sykes, G.M. and Matza, D. 'Techniques of neutralisation: a theory of delinquency', *American Sociological Review*, 1957, *22*, 664-70.
7. McCaghy, C.H. 'Drinking and deviance disavowal: the case of child molesters', *Social Problems*, 1968; *16*, 43-9.
8. Gelles, R.J., *The Violent Home: a Study of Physical Aggression Between Husbands and Wives*, Beverley Hills: Sage, 1974.
9. Coleman, D.H. and Strauss, M.A., 'Alcohol abuse and family violence' in *Alcohol, Drug Abuse and Aggression* (eds Gottheil, E., Druley, K.A., Skoloda, T.E. and Waxman, H.M.), Springfield, Illinois: Charles E. Thomas, 1983, pp. 104-24.
10. Box, S. *Power, Crime and Mystification*, London: Tavistock, 1983.
11. Levine, H.G., 'The good creature of God and the demon rum: colonial American and 19th-century ideas about alcohol, crime and accidents' in *Alcohol and Disinhibition: Nature and Meaning of the Link* (eds Room, R. and Collins, G.), Rockville, Maryland: National Institute on Alcohol Abuse and Alcoholism, 1983, pp. 111-61.
12. Winick, C., 'Drinking and disinhibition in popular culture' in *Alcohol and Disinhibition: Nature and Meaning of the Link* (eds Room, R. and Collins, G.), Rockville, Maryland: National Institute on Alcohol Abuse and Alcoholism, 1983, pp. 347-73.
13. Cohen, S., *Folk Devils and Moral Panics: The Creation of the Mods and Rockers*, Oxford: Martin Robertson, 1980.
14. Chibnall, S., *Law-and-Order News: An Analysis of Crime Reporting in the British Press*, London: Tavistock, 1977.
15. Hall, S., 'The treatment of 'football hooliganism' in the press' in *Football Hooliganism: The Wider Press and Media Context* (eds Ingham, R. *et al*), Inter-action Inprints: London, 1978.
16. Haralambos, M., *Sociology: Themes and Perspectives*, Slough: University Tutorial Press, 1980.
17. Montagu, A., *Learning Non-aggression: The Experience of Non-literate Societies*, Oxford: Oxford University Press, 1978.
18. Plant, M.A. 'Learning to drink' in *Alcoholism in Perspective* (ed. Grant, M.), London: Croom Helm, 1979.

19. Jahoda, G. and Cramond, J., *Children and Alcohol: A Developmental Study in Glasgow*, vol 1, London: HMSO, 1972.
20. Frude, N. and Gault, H. 'Children's understanding of aggression' in *Aggression and Violence* (eds Marsh, P. and Campbell, A.), Oxford: Blackwell, 1982.
21. Davies, J. and Stacey, B., *Teenagers and Alcohol: A Developmental Study in Glasgow*, vol 2. London: HMSO, 1972.
22. Robins, L., *Deviant Children Grown Up*, Baltimore: Williams & Wilkins, 1966.
23. Robins, L., 'A study of childhood predictors of adult anti-social behaviour: a replication from longitudinal studies', *Psychological Medicine*, 1978; *8*, 611-22.
24. West, D.J. and Farrington, D.P., *The Delinquent Way of Life*, London: Heinemann Educational, 1977.
25. Cline, H.F., 'Criminal behavior over the life span' in *Constancy and Change in Human Development* (eds Brim, O.G. and Kagan, J.), Cambridge, Massachusetts: Harvard University Press, 1980.
26. West, D.J., *Delinquency: Its Roots, Careers and Prospects*, London: Heinemann, 1982.
27. MacAndrew, C. and Edgerton, R.B., *Drunken Comportment: A Social Explanation*, London: Thomas Nelson & Sons Ltd., 1969.
28. Coid, J. '"Mania a potu:" a critical review of pathological intoxication,' *Psychological Medicine*, 1979; *9*, 709-19.
29. Marshall, M., *Weekend Warriors: Alcohol in a Micronesian Culture*, Palo Alto, California: Mayfield, 1979.
30. Feest, C.F., 'Notes on North American alcohol use' in *North American Indian Studies* (ed Hovens, P.), Gottingen, FRG: Edition Herodot, 1981.
31. Durkheim, E., *The Division of Labour in Society*, New York: Free Press, 1964.
32. Merton, R., *Social Theory and Social Structure*, New York: Free Press, 1957.
33. Horton, D., 'The functions of alcohol in primitive societies', *Quarterly Journal of Studies on Alcohol*, 1943, *4*, 292-303.
34. Field, P.B., 'A new cross-cultural study of drunkenness' in *Society, Culture and Drinking Patterns* (eds Pittman, D. and Snyder, C.), New York: John Wiley & Sons, 1962.
35. Levinson, D., 'Social setting, cultural factors and alcohol related aggression' in *Alcohol, Drug Abuse and Aggression* (eds Gottheil, E., Druley, K.A., Skoloda, T.E. and Waxman, H.M.), Springfield, Illinois: Charles C. Thomas, 1983, pp. 41-58.
36. Marsh, P., *Aggro: The Illusion of Violence*, London: Dent & Sons, 1978.
37. Marsh, P., Rosser, E. and Harre, R., *The Rules of Disorder*, London: Routledge & Keegan Paul, 1978.
38. Garbarino, M.S., *Sociocultural Theory in Anthropology: A Short History*, New York: Holt, Reinhart & Winston, 1977.
39. Wiles, P.N.P., 'Criminal statistics and sociological explanations of Crime' in *Crime and Delinquency in Britain*, (eds Carson, W.G. and Wiles, P.), Oxford: Martin Roberston and Co., 1971, pp. 174-91.
40. Herbert, D.T., 'Urban Crime: A geographical perspective' in *Social Problems and the City: Geographical Perspectives*, (eds Herbert, D.T. and Johnson, R.J.), Oxford: Oxford University Press, 1979, pp. 117-38.
41. Baldwin, J. and Bottoms, A., *The Urban Criminal: a Study in Sheffield*, London: Tavistock, 1976.
42. Rex, J. and Moore, R., *Race, Community and Conflict*, London: Oxford, 1967.

43. Gill, O., *Luke Street: Housing Policy, Conflict; and the Creation of the Delinquent Area*, London: Macmillan, 1977.
44. Harrison, P., *Inside the Inner City*, Harmondsworth, Middlesex: Penguin Books, 1983.
45. Murray, R. and Boal, F.W., 'The sociology of urban violence' in *Social Problems and the City: Geographical Perspectives* (eds Herbert, D.T. and Smith, D.M.), Oxford: Oxford University Press, 1983.
46. Lambert, J.R., *Crime, Police and Race Relations*, Oxford University Press: London, 1970.
47. McClintock, F.H., Avison, N.H., Savill, N.C. and Worthington, V.L., *Crimes of Violence*, London: Macmillan, 1963.
48. Graham, K., LaRocque, L., Yetmann, R., Ross, T.J. and Guistra, E., 'Aggression and barroom environments', *Journal of Studies on Alcohol*, 1980, *41*, 277-92.
49. Burns, T.F., 'Getting rowdy with the boys', *Journal of Drug Issues*, 1980, Spring, 273-86.
50. Wolfgang, M.E. and Ferracuti, F., *The Subculture of Violence: Towards an Integrated Theory in Criminology*, London: Tavistock, 1967.
51. Wolfgang, M.E., *Patterns in Criminal Homicide*, London: Oxford University Press, 1958.
52. Roizen, J., 'Alcohol and criminal behaviour among blacks: the case for research on special populations in *Drinking and Crime: Perspectives on the Relationships Between Alcohol Consumption and Criminal Behaviour*, (ed. Collins, J.J.), London: Tavistock Publications, 1982.
53. Lewis, O., *A Puerto Rican Family in the Culture of Poverty — San Juan and New York*, New York: Random House, 1966.
54. Robbins, R.H., 'Alcohol and the identity struggle: some effects of economic change on interpersonal relations' in *Beliefs, Behaviours, and Alcoholic Beverages: a Cross Cultural Survey* (ed Marshall, M.), Ann Arbor: University of Michigan Press, 1979.
55. Lurie, N.O., 'The world's oldest on-going protest demonstration: North American Indian drinking patterns', *Pacific Historical Review*, 1971, *40*, 311-22.
56. Toch, H., *Violent Men*, Chicago: Aldine, 1969.
57. Berkowitz, L., 'Violence and rule-following behaviour' in *Aggression and Violence* (eds Marsh, P. and Campbell, A.), Oxford: Blackwell, 1982.
58. Room, R., 'Alcohol and ethnography: A case of problem deflation?' *Current Anthropology*, 1984; *25*, 169-91.
59. Lang, A.R., 'Drinking and disinhibition: Contributions from psychological research' in *Alcohol and Disinhibition. Nature and Meaning of the Link* (eds Room, R. and Collins, G.), Rockville, Maryland: National Institute on Alcohol Abuse and Alcoholism, 1983, pp. 48-90.
60. Wilson, G.T., 'Alcohol and human sexual behaviour', *Behaviour Research and Therapy*, 1977, *15*, 239-52.
61. Feldman, M.P., *Criminal Behaviour: A Psychological Analysis*, London: John Wiley & Sons, 1977.
62. Coid, J., 'Alcoholism and Violence', *Drug and Alcohol Dependence*, 1982, *9*, 1-13.

8 ALCOHOL AND AGGRESSION — THE NATURE OF A PRESUMED RELATIONSHIP

Paul F. Brain

Introduction

This book re-examines, in a non-partisan manner, the thesis that acts of 'aggression' or violence can be caused by ingestion of alcohol. This is a view which has had a surprisingly wide currency amongst lay people, arbiters of public opinion and some policy makers. But how strong is the link between drinking and violence? We can, perhaps, best derive an answer to this question by examining the strands that are common to the diverse preceding chapters, and providing an overall conclusion.

A major reason for our inability to demonstrate *scientifically* a simple link between alcohol and violence, is that 'aggression' is by no means a heterogeneous entity.[1] As we have seen in Chapters 1 (especially), 4, 5, 6 and 7, this attribute consists of very diverse sets of phenomena in infra-human animals and man. Indeed, offence, defence or predation may be the predominant motivation involved in different situations where behaviour receives this label. Further, when using this terminology, we are often attaching our value-judgement of 'reasonableness' to the recorded action in that context (i.e. behaviour tends to be classed as aggression when, in the eyes of the observer, it represents an excessive or unjustified response to a set of circumstances). Consequently, on these grounds alone, a common underlying biological 'aggression substrate' which will be influenced by alcohol to generate reliable changes in behaviour, seems highly improbable. Indeed, one should note that aggression, like all behaviour, is essentially the result of a complex interplay between biological, situational and experiential factors.

As maintained in Chapter 2 by Berry and Brain, a major way in which alcohol may influence aggression is by modifying the activities of the neural and endocrine coordinating systems. These systems are interdependent, but may be considered separately for our ease of understanding. They note that in the brain, alcohol enters the lipid bilayer of nerve-cell membranes where it disrupts the constituent proteins which are important for normal neural activity. They emphasise that effects on particular proteins depend largely on their lipid environment. Indeed, a protein may have its functions increased by alcohol in certain cells whereas these activities are reduced or uninfluenced in the same substrate in other locations.

Berry and Brain also stress that there are no special targets or receptors for alcohol (unlike e.g. hormones, opiates and benzodiazepines). The non-specific membrane effects of alcohol consequently make it impossible to predict the effects of this compound on most neuronal properties. They note that this drug can increase *or* decrease: (a) the synthesis, storage, release and inactivation of central neurotransmitter substances (see also Chapter 3); (b) resting membrane potential and resistance; (c) neuronal excitability; and (d) post-synaptic receptor sensitivity. In each case only certain cells appear to be influenced, and different concentrations of alcohol may produce opposite effects. A further contrast with drugs that have specific targets is that one cannot directly reverse the neurophysiological effects of alcohol, although one may indirectly antagonise certain aspects of its actions. Berry and Brain suggest that an effective alcohol antagonist (an amethystic agent) would have to rapidly inactivate alcohol by 'binding' to it or quickly convert it to an inactive metabolite. Such considerations do highlight some of the difficulties of providing 'cures' for alcoholism.

Berry and Brain maintain that alcohol generally has a biphasic action on neuronal excitability (see some similar claims concerning behaviour in infra-human animals in Chapter 4). They note that low concentrations tend to increase this attribute whilst high concentrations, after transiently increasing it, progressively reduce excitability and spike amplitude. Impulse conduction is blocked only at lethal concentrations, which are consequently of little behavioural relevance. They note that alcohol seems to exert its main CNS effects by specific modulation of synaptic transmission rather than by a general depression of membrane responsiveness. Excitatory and inhibitory synapses may both be potentiated or depressed by this compound, again increasing the complexity of the situation.

It was also confirmed in Chapter 2 that the brain areas most intimately concerned with the expression of aggressive behaviour had been largely identified by brain stimulation studies.[2] The precise stimulation area appeared to determine whether the resulting attack was primarily concerned with offence, defence or predation (see also Chapter 1). In one system where it has been examined, alcohol increased the latency for cats to show stimulus-induced attack on an anaesthetised rat (NB it could be argued that this is predation rather than aggression). The drug produced problems of head-orientation and difficulties in jaw opening, but increased the force of biting shown by subjects. Low doses of alcohol are also said to potentiate affective defence ('sham rage') elicited by hypothalamic stimulation, whereas high doses depress such responses. Berry and Brain speculated that, as low doses increase and high doses decrease the amplitude of evoked hypothalamic potentials in response to stimulation of amygdaloid structures that facilitate affective defence, one may have a direct neurophysiological correlate of the biphasic effect of alcohol on behaviour. However, although certain neural areas appear capable of eliciting aggression under defined conditions, the brain has no single 'aggression centre'. Indeed, many interacting processes in the CNS appear to be non-specifically related to this behavioural category. Some of the variability of alcohol-induced effects on behaviour may be consequences of this lack of neural specificity and the relatively large impact of experience on such phenomena (which also produce varied results).

Berry and Brain emphasise that chronic consumption of alcohol often leads to tolerance to this drug: such effects can occur after even a single dose. They also record that neurophysiological and behavioural effects at a given blood-alcohol concentration may depend on whether the level is rising or falling. Berry and Brain note that full tolerance in mice takes about three days to develop and involves a number of adaptive changes by the brain to counter alcohol's deleterious effects. For example, several membrane changes occur, such as a reduction in the proportion of polyunsaturated fatty acids in the phospholipids of the synaptic membrane. On cessation of chronic drinking, the nervous system also takes time to readjust to the alcohol-free state. Amongst the withdrawal symptoms is an excited state which may be accompanied by aggressive episodes. Berry and Brain reviewed the evidence that chronic alcoholism may result in severe and possibly irreversible brain damage which could be responsible for violence in some clinical populations. They suggest that such damage may be caused by metabolites of alcohol (see Chapter 3) such as acetaldehyde or TIQs (reaction products of acetaldehyde and catecholamines which are formed in the brain and are related to the addictive opiate drugs). Indeed, it has been noted that TIQs increase alcohol preference in rats.

These authors note that a variety of neurotransmitter systems have been implicated in the modulation of aggressive behaviour[3] and all have been found to be modified by alcohol. They consequently opine that it is difficult to identify the specific systems involved in alcohol-induced changes in behaviour. Each type of 'aggression' seems to have its own multi-transmitter profile[4] and alcohol appears to alter the balanced manner in which they act.

Berry and Brain have shown that, like the brain, the endocrine system is highly integrated such that any deformation by alcohol is likely to have repercussions throughout the entire body. It consequently appears impossible to identify a single hormonal correlate of alcohol exposure that can be related to a behavioural change. Hormonal variation clearly influences aggressiveness and the signals that animals direct to each other, however, suggesting to these authors that behavioural endocrinology is likely to prove a promising approach in alcohol-aggression research. One should note, however, that the situation is complex, as hormones do not 'cause' behaviour, and the organism's activities can also modulate its hormonal secretion. Furthermore, different 'kinds' of aggression are influenced to variable degrees by particular hormonal profiles.[5,6]

Chapter 3 by Badawy also particularly emphasises the complex biochemical effects of alcohol on the organism, and makes the important point (also evident throughout this book) that the influences of this drug strongly depend on temporal factors. Not only does influence vary with time after administration, but acute effects of alcohol may be opposite to those seen after chronic exposure. He notes that alcohol withdrawal is also associated with its own array of phenomena. Badawy also stresses that ethanol's function as a toxic agent may involve disturbance of a wide variety of physiological processes in the liver (where this drug is mainly metabolised) and elsewhere in the body. Alcohol may exert its actions in a number of ways, but he particularly cites the widespread occurrence in the body of disturbances due to the metabolism of this drug (generating a variety of products; involving a number of enzyme systems and taking place in a wide range of locations). Evidence is provided that a spectrum of methodological variables (e.g. dose, species, age and sex) influence the precise metabolism of alcohol. Studies *in vitro* and *in vivo*, he notes, have confirmed that liver metabolism of ethanol is carried out by three main enzyme systems (alcohol dehydrogenase, catalase and the microsomal ethanol oxidising system). These seem to be of differing degrees of importance in different situations, but all oxidise ethanol to acetaldehyde. Acetaldehyde is further oxidised to acetate, largely by aldehyde dehydrogenase, and may serve as an energy substrate. Badawy emphasises that the relative activities of different enzyme systems can determine *how* the body reacts to alcohol.

Chapter 3 also stresses that alcohol uptake produces widespread disturbances in (especially) intermediary metabolism — in particularly changing metabolism of glucose, biogenic amines and hormones (see Chapter 2). Components of all these systems have been implicated in behavioural change, including aggression.[3,7,8,9,10] Badawy concentrates on the acute and chronic effects of ethanol on aspects of the synthesis, release and activities of e.g. GABA, catecholamines and serotonin. He notes that cerebral biogenic amine metabolism can be influenced by very low doses of ethanol in animals, suggesting that small amounts of alcoholic beverages can change both neurotransmission and behaviour. Obviously, dietary factors could also be of some importance here.[11] Badawy also suggests that although much work remains to be done on these complex relationships, there are indications that aggression generally appears *after* acute intake of an intoxicating dose of ethanol and during alcohol withdrawal, which are also times associated with changes in neurotransmitters.

Berry and Smoothy (Chapter 4) detail the effects of alcohol on aggression in a variety of infra-human vertebrates including fish, birds, rodents, cats, dogs and monkeys. They also emphasise the extraordinary range of tests that are said to assess this attribute. Their review confirms that all authorities agree that high doses of ethanol impair attack behaviour. They note, however, in contrast, that although some studies report that *low* doses of alcohol potentiate some aspects of aggressive behaviour, other workers find no such effects. They suggest that potentiations are likely to occur in timid or subordinate animals. The critical analysis by these authors reveals that a number of studies have produced 'successful' aggression-potentiating effects of aggression which are weak and/

or limited to restrictive aspects of the aggressive repertoire. Berry and Smoothy also suggest that moderate doses of alcohol can have marked anti-aggressive effects which are unassociated with obvious motor incapacitation. The same dose can, however, produce variable effects in different behavioural sub-types of animals (dominants, subordinates and fearful subjects). They also reveal that studies on the long-term effects of single doses of alcohol have failed to reveal potentiations of aggression in any species tested. They conclude that there is little evidence in this literature that alcohol directly stimulates aggression in animals, and potentiations (if they occur) are more likely to result from disinhibition (i.e. removal of a 'block' on such activities in experimentally suppressed subjects). Berry and Smoothy maintain that detailed analyses of behaviour are likely to generate more meaningful results in assessments of the pharmacological effects of alcohol (which can be very subtle). Indeed, ethological approaches enable one to be more certain of the specificity of alcohol's effects on behaviour.

Berry and Smoothy also suggest that alcohol increases timid/defensive activities in a number of situations, but leaves such behaviour largely unchanged in others. They also note that there is often a change in behaviour of non-treated animals towards alcohol-treated subjects. This may, in turn, alter the subject's aggressive responses. One should also consider the lasting effects of early exposure to this drug in animals. They note that the effects of prenatal exposure to alcohol have only been studied in rodents, where chronic application of low doses to pregnant animals tends to increase the potential for fighting in their offspring, an effect opposite to that achieved with high doses.

These authors also emphasise the importance of greater biochemical sophistication in studies assessing the effects of ethanol on animal behaviour. Blood-alcohol concentrations are rarely measured in alcohol-aggression experiments. Berry and Smoothy stress that such levels may depend, for example, on the route of administration, the time after application, the weight of the recipient and the subject's housing condition. Alcohol consumed by humans is contained in complex chemical solutions (e.g. beer, wine and vodka). These authors consequently suggest that the effects on behaviour of congeners which are found in beverage alcohols, should at least be considered. These factors have only been studied in fish, where they generally suppress aggression; but one cannot simply assume that all the effects of alcohol consumption are mediated by the substance's ethanol content.

Chapter 5 by Evans confirmed that alcohol has been frequently associated with a wide range of violent incidents in man. He notes that these have included homicide, felony, petty crime, sexual assault, violence within the family, and accidents. Evans concluded from the analysis of a variety of studies that there are many ways in which the data expressing the link between alcohol and violence could prove misleading. He suggests that the consumption of alcohol may be over- or under-reported as a result of bias inherent in the methods used to acquire that data. He also maintains that the way in which cases are processed by the police and the judicial system can distort the link between alcohol ingestion and subsequent behaviour. Furthermore, Evans claims that although all types of human violence have been associated with the consumption of alcohol, this is invariably with a *minority* of such cases. He suggests that alcohol is therefore only at best one of a number of 'causes' of violence in our species, the most important determinants of which are social and situational factors. Evans claims that alcohol-related violence is relatively rare in our society in relation to the man-hours spent drinking. This author suggests that the link between alcohol and violence is essentially a product of at least two types of phenomena. He is happy to assume that there is an acute pharmacological effect on behaviour, but feels that the association between chronic alcohol abuse and violence is unrelated to this former effect. Evans also suggests that the influence of alcohol on behaviour may be modified by social and environmental factors and (for the majority of people who drink) 'violence' is not the most likely outcome. It is also clear that the 'expectancy' effect (i.e. the response to the belief that one has consumed alcohol) on behaviour may be greater than the pharmacological impact of this drug.

Evans maintains (in Chapter 5) that there are always a number of plausible explanations for *any* link between the ingestion of alcohol and a category of human violence. He suggests that this drug may contribute to 'violence' in a number of ways. It may promote aggressiveness directly; it can increase risk taking, or it may simply interact with other drugs that influence behaviour. Evans feels that it is not yet clear whether alcoholism leads to violence or if excessive drinking and aggression are both symptoms of the same basic cause. He suggests, however, that some amelioration of alcohol-related crime is possible, and maintains that the identification of and treatment of alcohol abuse may be a cost-effective means of reducing recidivism in some 'habitual criminals'. He feels that such procedures may also produce other social benefits such as a decline in the suicide rate.

In Chapter 6, Coid (although discussing the matter rather differently from Evans in Chapter 5) also concludes that it is not possible to make accurate estimations of the various associations between alcohol and rape/sexual assault from available data due to the limitations of criminal statistics and the methodologies of previous research. He concludes that analysis of previous findings does not indicate major differences between rape situations where alcohol is present and those where it is absent. This drug can, however, he concludes, influence the offender's attitude and subsequent behaviour towards his victim, increasing the potential for violence and additional humiliation. Coid also believes that knowledge of the offender's alcohol intake can influence decision-making by justice personnel, as to the degree to which cases are 'founded' and the defendants convicted when the victim has been drinking. Experimental psychological research demonstrates the importance of 'expectation' to the drinker's subsequent behaviour, and suggests that alcohol may help to overcome factors that would normally render sexual assault less likely. Expectancy measured in the laboratory may be influenced, in turn, by societal attitudes to sexual and aggressive behaviour in drinkers. Decision-making by criminal justice personnel are said, by Coid, to be influenced by societal attitudes to women — particularly to women drinkers.

Chapter 7 of this book (also by Coid) examines an alternative approach to alcohol-related aggression in which socio-cultural factors are seen as the prime influences shaping this disinhibited behaviour. He feels strongly that the pharmacological properties of this drug cannot account for the wide repertoire of drunken behaviour seen in different locations, the changes seen in these locations over time, and the fact that disinhibition is not an inevitable consequence of drinking. Coid suggests that aggression is socially defined, and that the mere presence of alcohol can give aggressive behaviour a new social meaning. He maintains that individuals in society learn the social meanings of drinking and aggression at an early age, and that their attitudes and expectations are shaped by the culture that they belong to. Coid feels that researchers in this field are shifting from studies of tribal and non-industrialised societies to examine such socio-cultural theories in the urban setting. This author notes that, although the sociocultural perspective has been hailed by its advocates as a replacement for the earlier biological theories of alcohol-related aggression (with their attendant difficulties), this new approach also has inherent limitations.

This book consequently refutes the view that alcohol (via its effects on the brain especially) simply switches aggression on in humans and that such an interpretation is supported by experiments with a wide range of animals. The basic reason for this is that, although to the lay person, the question 'Does alcohol increase aggression?' sounds simple, there are a number of layers of complexity to this query which are apparent when one scientifically examines its components.

'Aggression' is a difficult term which is applied to an astoundingly varied group of activities and emotions. Indeed, the nature of this concept changes from authority to authority. Even activities which are superficially similar, in terms of the actions involved, may be viewed as appropriate (non-aggressive?) or inappropriate (aggressive?) by virtue of their context, the culture in which they occur, or the individual who performs them. One could maintain that there should be a strong imperative for scientists (and other authorities who influence perception of problems by the public) to minimise the use of the term 'aggression' as less value-laden terminologies are likely to create fewer problems. One may also argue that the rationale of studying 'aggression' out of its context (behaviour is a complex of changing activities that serve a variety of functions and express a number of needs and unequivocal aggression is often a very minor component in any behavioural encounter) is very dubious. Much can be said in favour of the new, more ethological approaches to the study of behaviour in laboratory animals, which attempt to record as many activities shown by the participants in a situation or encounter as is possible (further discussion on these considerations is provided in ref. 12). One should note, however, that this approach only provides one way of examining aggression and violence in humans. Human ethology generally involves an external observer recording the events in a short social encounter between other individuals, recommendedly in the manner of a Martian looking at an unknown terrestrial species (the problems and advantages of these approaches are discussed in ref. 13). In our species, changing (?) attitudes and popular perceptions (which may vary from culture to culture) can be at least as important to our understanding of the relationship between alcohol ingestion and violence. This is the essence of 'emic' approaches such as the socio-cultural analysis of human behaviour which has been used to provide an insight, for example, into phenomena such as 'football hooliganism'.[14] In such constructs, popular myths can be as important as real correlations. The impact of the environment on the expression of human 'aggression' has been considered elsewhere.[15] Alcohol could obviously be considered as both a component of the non-interpersonal environment *and* as a factor that is likely to influence human dialogue (in the most inclusive sense). In many situations one may need to consider the 'aggressor' (who doesn't always accept this label) and the 'victim' as components of a dynamic relationship. In addition to the material contained in this book, one may wish to refer to other considerations of aggression-alcohol relationships as studied in clinical situations. Rosenbaum *et al.*[16] have provided a very detailed account of their clinical experiences in a review which examines life events, stress and coping in alcoholic and violent patients; the neurophysiological assessments of violent and non-violent drinkers, Buss-Durkee hostility inventory scores in relation to drinking and violence, and (especially) considerations of 'battered women' in relation to these phenomena.

In addition, relating physiology to behaviour is never an easy process. Some of the difficulties of 'biological explanations' of human aggression have been reviewed elsewhere.[1] One must also emphasise that alcohol exerts extremely complex actions on physiology (there are often a wide range of potential indices of physiological change as well as there being a wide variety of inter-linked organ systems). A number of physiological processes may alter behaviour, e.g. changes in the function of the central nervous system or the activities of odour-producing glands may both change this attribute in monkeys and mice. The time-courses of these effects of ethanol are also crucial to our understanding of any obtained correlations. The influence of alcohol on biological systems is not only changed by prior exposure but factors such as an individual's expectancies (if an individual thinks he has been consuming alcohol, he often behaves as if he *has*). Ethanol may also change how experiences are perceived leading to modifications of *subsequent* behaviour. A further consideration emphasised in this volume is that traditional alcoholic beverages consumed by man contain a complex variety of substances (congeners and differing amounts of water as well as the ethanol), and physiological processes complicate this situation even more by rapidly generating a fluctuating array of metabolites. The potential behavioural influences of such factors has hardly been touched upon.

Having necessarily made all the above provisos, one should certainly *not* underplay the importance of considering the effects of alcohol (a rather ubiquitous, if socially acceptable drug in many societies) in human interactions incuding those receiving the attribute 'aggression'. The revealed complexities, rather than discouraging attempts to understand the link between alcohol and violence, should serve to stimulate a more sophisticated approach to this type of investigation. We should take on board our hard-gained understanding of the complexities inherent in behavioural terminology and description, and add to that our appreciation of the complex repercussions that follow exposing biological systems to alcohol. Unless we distance ourselves from the simple idea that alcohol 'causes' certain forms of activity, little meaningful progress will be made in this area. The association between alcohol and violence is a prime candidate for a truly multi-disciplinary effort, involving a successful 'marriage' between a variety of trusted behavioural approaches (which recognise the differences between species, cultures and individuals), and truly sophisticated biological investigation which does not concentrate on a single parameter and takes full account of the time dimension. Obviously, there is great scope for meaningful collaboration between behavioural scientists (from a variety of persuasions) and biologists who are attracted to interdisciplinary science.

References

1. Brain, P.F. 'Biological explanations of human aggression and the resulting therapies offered by such approaches: a critical evaluation' in *Advances in the Study of Aggression Volume 1* (eds Blanchard, R.J. and D.C.), New York: Academic Press, 1984, pp. 63-102.

2. Adams, D.B. 'Brain mechanisms for offense, defense and submission', *The Behavioral and Brain Sciences*, 1981, *2*, 201-41.

3. Valzelli, L. *Psychobiology of Aggression and Violence*, New York: Raven Press, 1981.

4. Daruna, J.H. 'Patterns of brain monoamine activity and aggressive behavior', *Neuroscience and Biobehavioral Reviews*, 1978, *2*, 101-13.

5. Brain, P.F. 'Hormones and aggression in infra-human vertebrates' in *The Biology of Aggression* (eds Brain, P.F., and Benton, D.), Alphen aan den Rijn: Sijthoff and Noordhoff, 1981, pp. 181-213.

6. Brain, P.F., Haug, M. and Kamis, A.B. 'Hormones and different tests for "aggression" with particular reference to the effects of testosterone metabolites' in *Hormones and Behaviour in Higher Vertebrates* (eds Balthazart, J., Prove, E., and Gilles, R.), Berlin: Springer-Verlag, 1983, pp. 290-304.

7. Benton, D., Kumari, N. and Brain, P.F. 'Mild hypoglycaemia and questionnaire measures of aggression', *Biological Psychology*, 1982, *14*, 129-35.

8. Brain, P.F. *Hormones and Aggression, Volume 1*, Montreal: Eden Press, 1977.

9. Brain, P.F. *Hormones and Aggression, Volume 2*, Montreal: Eden Press, 1978.

10. Brain, P.F. *Hormones Drugs and Aggression, Volume 3*, Montreal: Eden Press, 1979.

11. Eichelman, B., Elliot, G.R. and Barchas, J.D. 'Biochemical, pharmacological and genetic aspects of aggression' in *Biobehavioral Aspects of Aggression* (eds Hamburg, D.A. and Trudeau, M.B.), New York: Alan R. Liss Inc, 1981, pp. 51-84.

12. Brain, P.F. 'Comments on laboratory-based "aggression" tests', *Animal Behaviour*, 1984, *32*, 1256-7.

13. Brain, P.F. 'Classical ethology and human aggression' in *The Biology of Aggression* (eds Brain, P.F., and Benton, D.), Alphen aan den Rijn: Sijthoff and Noordhoff, 1981, pp. 603-23.

14. Marsh, P., Rosser, E. and Harre, R. *The Rules of Disorder*, London: Routledge & Kegan Paul, 1978.

15. Brain, P.F. 'Human aggression and the physical environment' in *Mental Health and the Environment* (ed. Freeman, H.L.), London: Churchill-Livingstone, 1985, pp. 97-120.

16. Rosenbaum, C.P., Adams, J.E., Scott, K.L., Renson, G.L., Tinklenberg, J.R. and Hanks, S.E. 'Alcohol and violence: a clinical study' in *Biobehavioral Aspects of Aggression* (eds Hamburg, D.A., and Trudeau, M.B.), New York: Alan R. Liss Inc., 1981, pp. 169-226.

INDEX

For Product Safety Concerns and Information please contact our EU representative GPSR@taylorandfrancis.com
Taylor & Francis Verlag GmbH, Kaufingerstraße 24, 80331 München, Germany

www.ingramcontent.com/pod-product-compliance
Ingram Content Group UK Ltd.
Pitfield, Milton Keynes, MK11 3LW, UK
UKHW022156190926
475702UK00003B/54
9781032610504